FEMALE SEXUALITY AND CULTURAL DEGRADATION IN ENLIGHTENMENT FRANCE

T0264896

In her study of eighteenth-century literature and medical treatises, Mary McAlpin takes up the widespread belief among cultural philosophers of the French Enlightenment that society was gravely endangered by the effects of hyper-civilization. McAlpin's study explores a strong thread in this rhetoric of decline: the belief that premature puberty in young urban girls, supposedly brought on by their exposure to lascivious images, titillating novels, and lewd conversations, was the source of an increasing moral and physical degeneration. In how-to hygiene books intended for parents, the medical community declared that the only cure for this obviously involuntary departure from the "natural" path of sexual development was the increased surveillance of young girls. As these treatises by vitalist and vitalist-inspired physiologists became increasingly common in the 1760s, McAlpin shows, so, too, did the presence of young, vulnerable, and virginal heroines in the era's novels. Analyzing novels by, among others, Jean-Jacques Rousseau, Denis Diderot, and Choderlos de Laclos, she offers physiologically based readings of many of the period's most famous heroines within the context of an eighteenth-century discourse on women and heterosexual desire that broke with earlier periods in recasting female and male desire as qualitatively distinct. Her study persuasively argues that the Western view of women's sexuality as a mysterious, nebulous force—Freud's "dark continent"—has its secular origins in the mid-eighteenth century.

Female Sexuality and Cultural Degradation in Enlightenment France

Medicine and Literature

MARY MCALPIN
University of Tennessee, USA

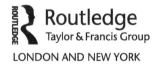

Routledge
Taylor & Francis Group

LONDON AND NEW YORK

First published 2012 by Ashgate Publishing

2 Park Square, Milton Park, Abingdon, Oxon OX14 4RN
711 Third Avenue, New York, NY 10017, USA

Routledge is an imprint of the Taylor & Francis Group, an informa business

First issued in paperback 2017

British Library Cataloguing in Publication Data
McAlpin, Mary, 1960–
Sexuality and cultural degeneration in Enlightenment France: medicine and literature.
   1. Literature and medicine – France – History – 18th century. 2. Literature and society – France – History – 18th century. 3. Literature and morals – History – 18th century. 4. Medical literature – France – History – 18th century. 5. French fiction – 18th century – History and criticism. 6. Young women in literature. 7. Sex in literature. 8. Precocious puberty – Social aspects – France – History – 18th century. 9. Enlightenment – France. 10. France – Social conditions – 18th century.
   I. Title
   840.9'3561'09033–dc23

Library of Congress Cataloging-in-Publication Data
McAlpin, Mary, 1960–
   Female sexuality and cultural degradation in enlightenment France: medicine and literature / by Mary McAlpin.
      p. cm.
   Includes bibliographical references and index.
   1. French literature—18th century—History and criticism. 2. Women in literature. 3. Sex in literature. 4. Literature and medicine—France—History—18th century. I. Title.
   PQ265.M33 2012
   840.9'005—dc23

                                                                 2011053307
ISBN 978-1-4094-2241-9 (hbk)
ISBN 978-1-138-11027-4 (pbk)

Contents

List of Figures

Acknowledgments

I would like to thank the University of Tennessee for supporting the writing of this book through two Summer Faculty Development Grants, a Professional Development Leave, and various other research related opportunities over the last six years. I would also like to thank the staff of the Bibliothèque Nationale in Paris for their generous help in locating documents. Various colleagues at the University of Tennessee read pieces of this study along the way, including the members of a reading group on the body and the Enlightenment sponsored by the U. T. Humanities Initiative: Misty Anderson, Lori Glover, and Denise Phillips. I would also like to thank Julia Douthwaite and Anne Vila for discussing this study with me, as well as the members of the Ancien Régime Group who read and responded to Chapter 5: Guillaume Ansart, Hall Bjørnstad, Jérôme Brillaud, Erec Koch, Suzanne Pucci, Jean-Luc Robin, and Holly Tucker. The anonymous Ashgate readers who responded so generously to this manuscript helped me to finalize my work and I thank them for their time while acknowledging that any remaining errors and infelicities are my own. Early versions of portions of Chapters 4, 5, and 6 appeared in *Studies in Eighteenth-Century Culture*, *Eighteenth-Century Studies*, and the *Journal of the History of Sexuality*, respectively, and I thank the editors and anonymous readers of those pieces for helping me to develop my work. Much love and thanks to Ray and to my beautiful daughter Celeste.

A Note on Translations and Scientific Texts

All translations from the French are mine, unless otherwise noted. I include below a list of the primary scientific texts cited in this study, in chronological order with titles translated into English (for the original French titles and full listings, consult the Bibliography). I also indicate if the author was associated with the Montpellier School of Medicine, when such information is available.

Buffon, *Natural History* (1749–1788). Buffon was a contemporary of the vitalists and his study of man as part of the animal kingdom was an important influence on their work.

Raulin, *On the Conservation of Children* (1749); *Treatise on White Flowers* (1766). Raulin was not directly associated with Montpellier, having earned his medical degree at Bordeaux. He built his career in Paris, where he specialized in the diseases of women.

Encyclopédie ou Dictionnaire raisonné des sciences, des arts et des métiers (1751–1765). Many of the medical and scientific articles in the *Encyclopédie* were written by vitalists or reflect vitalist theory.

Pomme, *Essay on the Vaporous Affections of the Two Sexes* (1760). Pomme is identified as a Montpellier doctor on the title page of his work; he earned a medical degree from Montpellier in the late 1750s.

Astruc, *Treatise on Women's Illnesses* (1761–1765). Astruc was one of the earliest and most famous of Montpelliervitalists; he held the Chair of Medicine at the Collège Royal in Paris from 1731 until his death in 1766.

Ballexserd, *Dissertation on the Physical Education of Children, From their Birth until the Age of Puberty* (1762). A Genevan physician, Ballexserd emphasized the reliance on natural processes that was central to the Montpellier movement.

Rousseau, *Emile, or On Education* (1762). As I argue in Chapter 1, the philosophy of Rousseau's famous pedagogical treatise relies heavily on the physiology of puberty.

Bienville, *Nymphomania* (1771). Little is known of Bienville, other than that he practiced medicine in Rotterdam and The Hague.

Goulin, *The Woman's Doctor* (1771). Despite Goulin's many publications, little is known of his life, including where he earned his medical degree.

Lignac, *On Man and Woman Considered Physically in the State of Marriage* (1772). Lignac's title page indicates that he was a surgeon.

Le Moré, *Institutional Principles or How to Raise Children* (1774). Le Moré was also the author of a book aimed at helping young children learn history.

Roussel, *Physical and Moral System of Woman* (1775). Roussel was a physician at Montpellier and is closely associated with the promulgation of vitalist theories on women.

Virard, *Essay on the Health of Nubile Girls* (1776). Virard was a doctor at the University of Montpellier; the *Essay* was republished in French in 1779 and again in an Italian translation in 1794.

Daignan, *Tableau of the Varieties of Human Life* (1786). Daignan's title page identifies himself as a "Montpellier doctor."

Bressy, *Research on the Vapors* (1789). Bressy's title page identifies him as a doctor at the University of Montpellier.

Ferrier, *On Puberty Considered as the Crisis of Childhood Maladies* (1799). A dissertation for the Montpellier School of Medicine.

Cabanis, *On the Relations between the Physical and the Moral Aspects of Man* (1802). An ideologue and a Paris physician, Cabanis lavishly praised the Montpellier legacy.

Moreau de la Sarthe, *Natural History of Woman* (1803). Moreau de la Sarthe studied and made his career in Paris; his treatise reprises a host of vitalist observations about women.

Introduction:
Daughters of Eve

It does not suffice to speak of women, and to do it well, Thomas; make me see them. Suspend them in front of my eyes like so many thermometers marking the slightest vicissitudes in mores and usages.

—Denis Diderot, "On Women"

Among the more persistent tenets of the history of ideas is the belief that Enlightenment-era intellectuals universally embraced the theory of mankind's innate perfectibility.[1] The present study joins a critical conversation on this supposed hubris by examining a related discourse among eighteenth-century cultural philosophers: the belief that European civilization faced an imminent and catastrophic collapse due to the physical and moral degradation of its citizens.[2] The underlying assumption was that although Europeans had indeed advanced to a dizzying level of human social organization by virtue of their superior inventiveness and energy, this attractive exterior hid a slowly spreading "disease" that would soon bring about a catastrophic breakdown. This discourse of imminent regression was particularly prevalent in France, where it achieved the level of a cultural commonplace. The prescribed "cure" was primarily medical in nature and involved a revolution in hygiene designed to stave off the negative effects of the civilized state while preserving its benefits. The goal was not a return to "the state of nature," but rather the amelioration of the degraded bodies and minds of urban residents attainable only by following nature's precepts.

In the following pages, I explore a central component of this battle against degradation: the assumption that the principal cause of this collapse was the premature awakening of sexual desire in young girls. I focus primarily on two cultural manifestations of this belief, the medical (Chapters 1 and 2) and the literary (Chapters 3, 4, and 5). I begin with the appearance in the 1760s of a new genre, the adolescent hygiene treatise, designed to instruct parents in how to shepherd their offspring through the difficult "revolution" of puberty. These treatises brought together a number of the key components of Montpellier vitalism, and many, although not all, were written by physicians associated with the Montpellier School of Medicine. The vitalists viewed puberty as the moment at which previously "identical" children were "born" or "awakened" to sex, by

---

[1]   Most famously expressed in Max Horkheimer and Theodore Adorno's *Dialectic of Enlightenment* (1944).

[2]   Alexandre Wenger places the origins of this obsession in George Cheyne's 1733 *The English Malady, or, a Treatise of Nervous Diseases* (*La Fibre littéraire: Le Discours médical sur la lecture au XVIIIᵉ siècle* [Geneva: Droz, 2007], 207).

virtue of the fluids released into their bodies by their genitals at this period of physical and moral crisis. Temperament (overall health), the parents who read these treatises learned, was fixed only when the transformation wrought by the pubescent years was completed and the young person's body stabilized. Keeping one's child safe from negative influences during this period was crucial to ensuring the future production of his or her own healthy offspring. The continuation of the family line was at stake—not to mention the future of European civilization.

These treatises were novel in many ways. Written in French for a popular audience, rather than in the Latin traditionally used for medical texts, they addressed sexuality in a decidedly secular tone and presented adult sexual intercourse (between heterosexuals and within marriage) as healthy and necessary, not only for the population as a whole but also for individual men and women. This celebration of human sexual desire was complicated in the case of adolescent girls by the dangers said to be posed by premature "knowledge" of sexuality. The danger for prepubescent girls was the eruption of early puberty due to exposure to lascivious influences, but even girls going through puberty had to be carefully protected in order to keep them quite thoroughly ignorant of the sexual nature of the (quite powerful) physical stirrings they were said to be experiencing. Only when their wombs were "fully formed" were they to be enlightened (by the events of the wedding night) as to what their bodies were said to crave so desperately. Adolescent boys were also said to be in need of protection from the cultural forces at work upon them, although they were presented as by no means as vulnerable as their female counterparts to such influences as novels, sensual images, and suggestive conversations.

As these treatises illustrate with particular force, the ripe young virgin and her vulnerable innocence, always a richly evocative type, took increasing hold of the French cultural imagination as the eighteenth century progressed.[3] As Diderot's reference to women as "cultural thermometers" indicates, the belief that the highly suggestive nature of women made them a clear reflection of cultural morality is a common theme in this period, made explicit in a number of philosophical texts that I examine alongside the hygiene treatises in Chapters 1 and 2. I turn to literary manifestations of this theme in Chapters 3, 4, and 5. Young women and the dangers they faced on entering society was a dominant theme in this era's most popular novels. I refer to this literary type as the "ingénue," for as in the medical treatises, her liminal status as both child and woman—reflected in her ignorance of the nature of the physical desires she both inspires and experiences— is the essence of her fictional identity. The symbolic status of the postpubescent

---

[3]   Nadine Berenguier cites the eighteenth-century focus on adolescence in her study of Mme de Graffigny's *Letters of a Peruvian Woman* (1747): "The increased consciousness of the educational needs of adolescent girls, born at a point when written culture was on the rise, engendered not only many works in which women's education was debated, but also a number of manuals written specifically for women" ("Zilia, une adolescente hors du commun," *SVEC* 2004:12, 312–13).

virgin made her ideally suited to the fictional exploration of certain compelling eighteenth-century social issues surrounding marriage, sexuality, religion, gender politics, and motherhood. While I examine a number of novels and essays in passing, I am especially interested in works by Jean-Jacques Rousseau, Choderlos de Laclos, and Marie-Jeanne Roland, for each of these authors uses the figure of the ingénue to explore the commonplace of cultural degradation. The result is a revealing mirror of the eighteenth-century cultural imagination.

The Ingénue in Enlightenment Thought

The ingénue is the trope of choice for the ambiguities associated with Enlightenment philosophy in that she is such a compelling mix of qualities: beautiful, desirable, desiring, yet in her ignorance highly dangerous not only to herself but to her society as a whole. She embodies the dialectic at the anxious core of Enlightenment debates on the nature of the human, for she participates in both sides of the contradictory pairings at the heart of eighteenth-century cultural theory: nature and civilization, on the one hand, and degradation and perfectibility, on the other. Her use as a figure of general cultural anxiety is perhaps most clearly expressed in the paintings of one of the era's most influential artists, Jean-Baptiste Greuze. "The Broken Jug" is one of Greuze's most famous works, so much so that his gravesite in the Montparnasse Cemetery in Paris includes a life-size sculpture based on this painting: a young, beautiful girl holding a large jug with a conspicuous hole.[4] The sculptor could not reproduce the most important aspect of the painting for my purposes, for while the girl's body is prominently foregrounded by Greuze, the background contains both trees (perhaps meant to indicate a country setting) and an antique fountain.

The girl's dress seems hardly appropriate to the task of gathering water in the countryside, and indicates that her symbolic status is far more general than a reference to the topos of the innocent village girl exposed by her daily tasks to the wiles of far more sophisticated men. The fountain's decorations also seem to indicate that more is at stake than a reference to the old French saying "the pitcher goes to the well so often that at last it is broken" (*tant va la cruche à l'eau qu'à la fin elle se casse*). The antique motif may be a symbolic reference to decline and ruin; more certain is that its sad-eyed lion, spouting water from its mouth, reflects the loss of innocence just experienced by the young girl. The breast she makes no effort to cover is a symbol of her fallen state rather more dramatic than the lion or the jug itself, placed in the shadows to the bottom left of the painting.

---

[4]   There were at least three versions of this painting; the Louvre dates its version to 1771. For more on Greuze, see Anita Brookner, *Greuze: The Rise and Fall of an Eighteenth-Century Phenomenon* (Greenwich, CT: New York Graphic Society, 1972); for more on sexual themes in eighteenth-century painting, see Philip Stewart, "Sexual Encoding in Eighteenth-Century Literature and Art," *Sexuality and Culture* 8.2 (Spring 2004): 3–23.

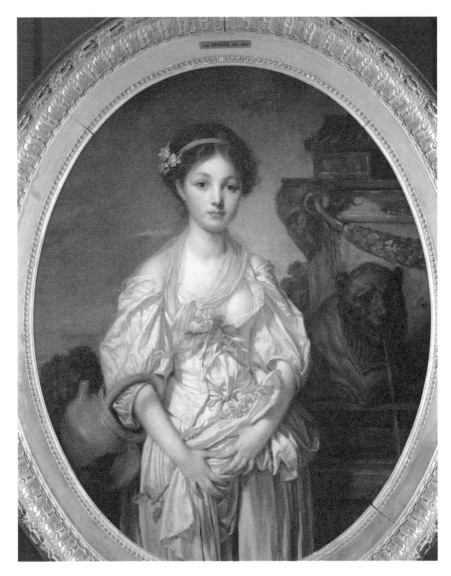

Fig. I.1   Jean-Baptiste Greuze (1725–1805). "The broken jug," 1772–1773.
The Louvre. Photograph © Erich Lessing/Art Resource, NY.

Another indication of this "loss" reveals rather a gain: the young woman directs her eyes squarely at the viewer, in contrast to the lowered gaze of the (much later) statue.[5] Greuze has represented, in this painting said to have been commissioned by Mme du Barry, much more than the mere loss of innocence said to accompany defloration. He has also portrayed the sharp and sudden gain in rationality said to accompany this "loss," both in the folklore and the medical theories of the day, as I go on to explore below. While I will only occasionally turn to paintings as artistic expressions of the cultural value of the eighteenth-century ingénue, given that written representations offer much more detail, it is important to note at the beginning of this study the impossibility of separating eighteenth-century writers into such delineated categories as "novelist," "physiologist," "political theorist," or "philosopher." Authors such as Rousseau, Diderot, and Laclos obviously considered themselves quite capable of writing on physiological topics and of popularizing their scientific opinions in a variety of genres, and even the most medically focused of the treatise writers whose works I examine create strikingly novelistic tableaux in their writings, designed to touch the hearts of their readers and render the works' prescriptions all the more compelling.

The widespread emphasis on the dramatic physical and moral consequences of the premature sexualization of young girls that arose in the middle of the eighteenth century is tied to a number of important changes in the philosophy of the self during this period. In addition to the increasing secularization of eighteenth-century French culture, one of the most important philosophical shifts in this regard is the rise of a rhetoric of sexual incommensurability. While Michel Foucault famously situated the medicalization of sexuality in the late eighteenth and early nineteenth centuries, scholars such as G. S. Rousseau have argued that sexology as a science has its origins in the mid-eighteenth century.[6] With the decline of the influence of the Church on scientific writing, those thoughts and acts previously placed under the rubric of sexual "deviance" and simply condemned could be addressed in an objective, scientific manner not possible in previous eras. This insight has been crucial to recent work on the history of Enlightenment sexuality, particularly with regard to the attacks on male masturbation and homosexuality that arose and proliferated during the eighteenth century.

I argue that the need to maintain unmarried girls in a state of sexual ignorance was an equally significant cultural effect of this emerging scientific discourse. The virtuous "new man" of the Enlightenment, soon to develop into the *citoyen* of the Revolutionary imagination, was partnered with a "new woman" whose virtue was seen as even more crucial to a well-functioning society than that of her male partner. And just as the condemnation of masturbation and homosexuality remained firmly in place despite the newly scientific approach to such "deviant"

---

[5] The sculptor is Ernest Dagonet, 1856–1926.

[6] "Cette mutation se situe au tournant du XVIIIe et du XIXe siècle; elle a ouvert la voie à bien d'autres transformations, qui en dérivent" (Michel Foucault, *La Volonté de savoir*, in *Histoire de la sexualité* [2 vols, Paris: Gallimard, 1976], I:155).

behaviors, there was much that was "old" about the new woman. Her status as a far less rational and thus far more dangerous creature than her male counterpart was the most striking attribute she shared with her pre-Enlightenment foremothers. The "dangers" attached to the sexuality of attractive young women remained firmly in place, in other words, although the blame shifted from their "frail" shoulders to those of their parents. This reconceptualized woman was very much the secular "daughter of Eve," recast as vulnerable by virtue of her particular physiological organization rather than dismissed as a willfully sinful creature, but occupying the same symbolic role. Diagnosing women as the principal cause of the problems in what should have been the Eden of the civilized lifestyle meant that controlling their behavior was key to ameliorating the lives of men. By the end of the century, the need to relegate all women to the private sphere of home and motherhood, for the good of society, was a firmly ensconced Republican value. As Londa Schiebinger succinctly puts the matter: "After the 1750s the anatomy and physiology of sexual difference seemed to provide a kind of bedrock upon which to build relations between the sexes. The seemingly superior build of the male body (and mind) was cited more and more often in political documents to justify men's social dominance."[7]

There were, of course, competing, protofeminist philosophies of "femaleness" in existence from mid-century onward, but the rise of radical sexual differentiation both reflected and influenced profound changes in the era's philosophical and medical discourse. Consider the title of the famous defense of women's intellect by the seventeenth-century Cartesian philosopher François Poullain de la Barre: *On the Equality of the Two Sexes, A Physical and Moral Discourse in Which We See the Importance of Abandoning One's Prejudices* (1673). The discourse in question is declared both "physical and moral," but these two realms are not indissociably linked for de la Barre, as they will be by the middle of the eighteenth century in most considerations of woman's intellect. Liselotte Steinbrügge observes that de La Barre wrote with a fundamentally different philosophical viewpoint than these later authors: "[For Poullain de la Barre and his followers], woman's biological nature had played only an insignificant role in regard to her intellectual capabilities, because, in the Cartesian tradition, they gave precedence to reason, which they conceived of as genderless. Thomas and Roussel, in contrast proceeded from woman's physiological constitution in order to determine her intellectual capacity."[8]

The references given are to the *Essay on the Character, Mores, and Mind of Women in Different Centuries* (1772) by the poet, critic, and Academician Antoine-Léonard Thomas, and to the *Physical and Moral System of Woman* (1775) by Pierre Roussel, a Montpellier-trained physiologist. The disparate professions of

---

[7]   Londa Schiebinger, *The Mind Has No Sex? Women in the Origins of Modern Science* (Cambridge, MA: Harvard University Press, 1989), 216.

[8]   Liselotte Steinbrügge, *The Moral Sex: Woman's Nature in the French Enlightenment* (New York: Oxford University Press, 1995), 36.

these two figures illustrates how commonplace the assumption of an indissociable and highly sexed mind–body connection had become by the latter half of the eighteenth century. Roussel's work is in many ways the acme of the many medical treatises on this topic, and the following declaration from the *Physical and Moral System of Woman* is frequently cited to illustrate the insistence on differentiation during this time: "Woman is woman not only in one place, but in every respect from which she may be viewed."[9] While Roussel does go on to acknowledge (citing Hippocrates) that the differences between men and women may at times be "the effect of education and manner of life," he insists that there is a radical, innate difference between the sexes present in all countries and all peoples, a universal sexual binarism such that while some men are stronger than other men, they are in all cases stronger than their female counterparts (16). As for perfectibility, Michael Winston notes of Roussel's philosophy: "Unlike Helvétian or Buffonian views of progress, whereby all humans are theoretically capable of improvement, only the man possesses the physiological attributes necessary to advance in Roussel's system."[10]

This radically new philosophy of sexual differentiation was in great part the product of Roussel's predecessors at the Montpellier School of Medicine. The historian of science Elizabeth A. Williams gives a useful and telling definition of "physiology" as it is best understood in this vitalist theoretical context: "The primordial law of organized beings was that they lived and functioned by virtue of the interconnected activities of the 'animal economy,' which was empowered by some kind of vital force or forces. Thus physiology was the study of the interrelated, systemic, harmonious operations that simultaneously manifested and sustained the life of bodies that enjoyed vitality."[11] The vitalists were explicitly anti-Cartesian in their emphasis on moral determinism, and this insistence on the inseparability of mind and body, alongside the variability at the heart of the vitalist vision of the human body, led to two important "discoveries," as I explore in depth in Chapter 1. The first is related to the centrality of variability to vitalist thought, and declares that sexual differentiation begins only at puberty. The second concerns the outcome of the "revolution" of puberty, for this process is said to produce, in the case of young women, soft-brained individuals whose characteristically fluid minds and bodies are highly susceptible to outside stimuli. While the treatises stress that developing young men must avoid masturbation and the accompanying loss of semen or risk their own mental and physical perversion, young girls are granted far more attention, given that their hypersensitivity to external influences

---

9 Pierre Roussel, *Système physique et moral de la femme* (Paris: Vincent, 1775), 2. Future references in the text.

10 Michael E. Winston, *From Perfectibility to Perversion: Meliorism in Eighteenth-Century France* (New York: Peter Lang, 2005), 104.

11 Elizabeth A. Williams, *The Physical and the Moral: Anthropology, Physiology, and Philosophical Medicine in France, 1750–1850* (Cambridge: Cambridge University Press, 1994), 11.

is said to make them less resistant to the negative cultural forces at work upon their physico-moral constitutions. As a result, young women are portrayed as the unwitting bellwethers of a generalized cultural decline, and the surveillance of their sexual innocence is cast as absolutely essential to the production of future generations of healthy citizens.

The supposed rapid increase in gynecological diseases among young girls and women is often cited in the hygiene treatises as evidence of the degeneration said to accompany the overly civilized lifestyle, with "white flowers" identified as one of the most noxious of such illnesses (from the Latin *fluor albus*, or "white flow"; it is now known as *leucorrhaea*). As I examine in Chapter 2, a young woman suffering from such a disease was said to be a grave danger to society as a whole. She was declared unsuitable for marriage, given that she might infect her husband, might be sterile, or worse yet, might produce weak, feeble-minded offspring. A number of recent studies have taken up the related topic of meliorism, understood as the Enlightenment project of improving or perfecting man that culminates in the Revolutionary vision of the "new man," capable of taking on responsibility for his own destiny (a republican destiny, needless to say). But while I rely on these studies to a degree, I stand apart from the work of scholars interested in the overall theme of meliorism and its nineteenth-century successor, eugenics, in that I am interested in the "new woman" of eighteenth-century political rhetoric in her most essentialized, medicalized configuration.[12] Her role as companion to a newly revitalized European man interests me less than what she as a specific cultural trope expresses about the cultural conflicts and anxieties of her time, that led to the ideal of a female creature destined to domestic confinement and quite excluded from civil (political) affairs and responsibilities.

I devote Chapters 3 and 4 to an examination of two of the most influential fictional considerations of eighteenth-century womanhood, both published during the height of the popularity of the hygiene treatises of interest to me. In Chapter 3, I consider the century's best-selling novel, Rousseau's *Julie, or The New Heloise* (1761) in conjunction with his highly influential pedagogical treatise *Emile, or On Education* (1762). As I argue in Chapter 1, *Emile* is an early example of the type of treatise on childhood hygiene that interests me, in that the physiology of puberty plays a powerful role in determining how this young boy and his future wife, Sophie, are to be educated. I place the transcendent virtue of Julie, one of

---

[12]   One can see the transformation from hygiene to eugenics in the work of Pierre-Jean-Georges Cabanis, the well-known ideologue physician and an admirer of the vitalists: "Hygiene must aspire to perfect the general nature of man ... It is time, and in many other fields as well, to act systematically in a manner worthy of this period of regeneration" (*Rapports du physique et du moral de l'homme*, 2 vols, Paris: Crapart, Caille, and Ravier: An X [1802]), I:481–2. Studies of the nineteenth-century pseudo-science of eugenics that draw on eighteenth-century medical sources include Anne Carol, *Histoire de l'eugénisme en France. Les médecins et la procréation, XIXᵉ–XXᵉ siècles* (Paris: Seuil, 1995). The principal eighteenth-century work referenced in this debate is Charles Augustin Vandermonde's *Essai sur la manière de perfectionner l'espèce humaine* (1756).

the era's most beloved fictional characters, in the context of the (only apparently) contradictory treatment of Sophie in order to argue that Rousseau's vision of women, heavily inflected by climate theory and other physiological concerns, is far less out of step with the sexual politics of his day than has been generally accepted. While not as closely associated with vitalist philosophy as Diderot, Rousseau was taken seriously by the authors of the many treatises on adolescent hygiene who succeeded him. What perhaps most distinguishes Rousseau is the wide range of his scientific arguments; he can be claimed for natural history writing as easily as I am associating him with the physiology of puberty.[13]

Choderlos de Laclos's philosophy of female sexuality is the subject of Chapter 4. His *Dangerous Liaisons* (1782) occupies an important place in my study as an example of the evolution of the physiological discourse in the novel after Rousseau. I argue that Laclos's complex cast of female characters, carefully placed at different stages of innocence and degradation, are to be understood as expressions of his unique theory of woman's role in civilized society. This theory of sexuation and cultural degradation is found in an essay contemporary to Laclos's novel, "On Women and Their Education" (1783), a piece that like *Emile* is best read as a physiological treatise. In this essay, rather than focusing on the practicalities of educating women, Laclos indicts his society and calls upon French women to return to what they have lost, at least to the extent that this regression is possible. To demonstrate what was lost, Laclos describes in detail how a young girl would have come to puberty and thus sexuality in the state of nature. This young woman's free, promiscuous life is then contrasted to the constrained, joyless existence of eighteenth-century French women.

Laclos nevertheless conforms to the physiological givens of his day, in that while he blames the civilized lifestyle for putting women in the position of needing men, he advises his female counterparts to be so many virtuous Julies in order to attract and fix the best available male protector. By placing Laclos's essay and novel alongside the work of other authors who argue that woman's innate sexuality is best expressed in a monogamous and fairly limited life at home as a wife and mother, I move my study toward my final chapter, a consideration of the Revolutionary ethos of femininity. The vitalist theories of female sexuality, as popularized by their hygiene treatises, played a key role in this developing philosophy of womanhood. That male sexuality and morality were also fully determined by materialist causes, according to this theory of sexual bifurcation, was countered by the notion that men's bodies were far less susceptible to outside influences. Men could thus be said to remain the thinking masters of their cultural situation, as Steinbrügge writes:

> The eighteenth century is the period when the sex-specific character attributed to
> men and women developed and diverged; it is the epoch in which the ideological
> and institutional foundations were laid for women's exclusion from civil rights

---

[13] See Mark Hulling, *The Autocritique of Enlightenment: Rousseau and the Philosophes* (Cambridge, MA: Harvard University Press, 1994), 172.

and higher education—in short, from public life. It is the age that saw the
emergence of an image of female nature that allowed precisely these exclusions
to be considered 'natural.'[14]

I end this study in Chapter 5 with a consideration of how one woman negotiated
this exclusion by examining the first modern autobiography by a French woman,
Marie-Jeanne Roland's *Private Memoirs* (1795). By century's end, I argue, the
established vision of "natural" female sexuality had come to consist of a dichotomy
of modesty and vanity. "Modesty" is to be understood quite technically as an innate
resistance on the part of women to engage in sexual activity, a resistance intended,
by nature, to arouse men. Female vanity is then defined as a complementary yet
contrary urge: the equally innate desire on the part of women to attract men.
These competing instincts are said to produce the "dance" so often described in
eighteenth-century works on sexuality in the state of nature, a dance in which
natural woman is said to lead. She begins by casting teasing looks, then flees
after attracting the attention of her chosen mate. After he pursues and captures his
fleeing "prey," the two experience mutual satisfaction and part, perhaps never to
see each other again. Civilized women are of course said to have "gone beyond"
this easy reconciliation of their opposing instincts, and are indeed presented as
caught in an impossible double bind, by which any display of sexual aggression
leads to the accusation of lasciviousness, while the refusal of male sexual advances
opens women to the label "prude" or "coquette."

Roland's negotiation of this contradiction at the heart of eighteenth-century
discourse on female virtue is all the more revealing in that she was a student, indeed
an amateur practitioner, of medicine. Roland's astonishingly open treatment in her
Private Memoir of an incident of sexual abuse that she experienced at age ten
and of her subsequent, triumphant passage through the "revolution" of puberty
are informed by a close knowledge of both the physiological and the fictional
works of her day. In a work begun in the prisons of the Terror and left unfinished
at her execution, and clearly designed to answer her many detractors in the
Revolutionary press, Roland provides a self-justification that also constitutes an
insight into how women intellectuals reacted to the "new woman" envisioned by
the vitalists. Her work is all the more valuable in that rather than contesting this
vision of womanhood, she adopts its core principles to her own ends.

Montpellier Vitalism and the Discovery of Sex

A preliminary introduction to the Montpellier vitalists and their philosophy of
medicine is necessary in order to place the hygiene treatises, novels, and other
writings that I consider in the following chapters in historical context. In the
second part of this introduction, I consider two key principles linked to the vitalists'
"discovery" of femaleness: first, the reunification of the physical and the moral, in

---

[14]   Steinbrügge, *The Moral Sex*, 4.

opposition to Cartesian dualism; and second, the importance of climate theory, or environmental determinism, to their theories of cultural degradation.

The term "vitalism" is of course not limited to the Montpellier school, but is rather applied to any system of thought, such as that of Galen and, more influentially still, Aristotle, that privileges vital forces in living organisms over purely mechanical explanations of the life processes. In order to understand Montpellier vitalism, one needs a basic understanding of mechanism, the theory of the human organism, in opposition to which the Montpellier vitalists developed their own, highly influential vision of human physiology. The mechanist view of the human organism begins with the rejection of Galenic humoralism, a view of the body formulated in the second century by Galen of Pergamon and much influenced by Hippocratism. Galenists envisioned the body as an inert structure animated by spirit-filled fluids, or humors, a view that in the wake of the New Science developed in the late seventeenth century came to be viewed as hopelessly outdated. The mechanists argued that far from comprising a static container for the all-important humors, the bones and other "hard" structural parts were the engines of the bodily functions, working just like a set of pumps and presses on the glands and organs to produce, expel, and control the flow of liquids.

The philosophies of medicine with which mechanism is most intimately linked are iatrophysics and iatrochemistry, more generally known as iatromechanics. These labels cover the common theories of physicians (*iatro*) who, inspired by Cartesianism and Newtonianism, saw physical (muscle action, etc.) or chemical processes as central to the fundamental nature of life. The most "mechanical," as well as the most influential, of these late seventeenth- and early eighteenth-century physiologists was Hermann Boerhaave (1668–1738), Chair of Medicine at the University of Leiden from 1701 until his death. Boerhaave promoted a view of health based on hydrostatics, or the balance of pressures, in a body viewed as a system of interacting, interdependent liquids and solids, and defined health as the maintaining of a balance, or proper level, of pressure.[15]

As the continuing importance of fluids to this description of bodily functions illustrates, as well as the importance of "balancing" the different liquids, humoralism was never rejected wholesale by mechanists but was rather reincorporated into a system that emphasized different components of the bodily system. But unlike the proponents of the coming vitalist revolution in medical theory, there was for Boerhaave and his many disciples nothing inherently mysterious about the humors nor about the bodily functions in general, however complex they might be. The fluids and solids acted together in a logical manner, with the transcendent soul as the separate, animating force. Any remaining "secrets" of the body's mechanics would be clearly revealed to the scientist who had the training and took the time necessary to uncover them. Dissection was the tool of choice for such discoveries,

---

[15] See G. A. Lindeboom, *Herman Boerhaave: The Man and His Work* (London: Methuen, 1968).

and its practice allowed an extraordinary acceleration of anatomical knowledge in a relatively short period of time.

Boerhaave's influence started to wane in the 1730s when a group of like-minded doctors associated with the Montpellier School of Medicine began to question the Cartesian view of the machine body as animated by a separate soul. In doing so, they were challenging scientific assumptions that were no longer "new," but rather quite solidly established. They contested the mechanical explanation that the fluids were moved about (controlled) by the muscles and bones, proposing instead, as had Galen, that the body's complex systems were managed by the innate (vital) forces present in these fluids. They went far beyond Galenic physiology however, for the invasive investigations of the mechanists had demonstrated that the body was no mere sack filled with humors, but was rather a complex combination of systems (circulatory, nervous, etc.) through which the bodily fluids moved—or from the mechanist point of view, were moved—in a precise, regulated manner. Rather than merely resurrecting Galenism per se, the vitalists combined this ancient view of the body with the new knowledge gained by the mechanist focus on dissection. The vitalist theory of physiology did however recast the muscles and bones as inert structures, serving at best as something of a shell or scaffolding designed to support the real work of the organs and their specialized humors. Most importantly, the vitalists placed the brain (and thus the mind) under the control of liquids secreted by organs, leading to a vision of the "soul" that was quite material.[16]

The vitalist rejection of Cartesian dualism was thus not without political consequences, for the vitalist vision of the mind and body as fundamentally interconnected and mutually dependent pointed toward moral determinism, in direct contradiction to Church dogma. While the move toward overt secularism in the writings of eighteenth-century scientists constitutes a major moment in the history of ideas, it is important to note, as does Daniel Mornet, that the majority of natural historians active during this period were engaged in attempting to accord their observations with the literal word of scripture.[17] Although it is easy to underestimate the extent to which Cartesian dualism had itself constituted a break with Church doctrine, dualism had allowed the mechanists to stay safely within the boundaries of a number of important ecclesiastical dictates, such as free will and the superiority of the human over the animal.[18] By the early eighteenth

---

[16]   Whether or not any of the vitalists should be placed squarely under the philosophical label "materialist" is a complex question; I will merely cite Jean Ehrard, who remarks that in spite of the occasional exception such La Mettrie's infamous *Man a Machine* (1747), "The most characteristic trait of the mid-century was not a penchant for extreme attitudes, but to the contrary the flight from destructive choices" (*L'Idée de nature en France dans la première moitié du XVIIIe siècle*, 2 vols [Paris: S.E.V.P.E.N, 1963], I:197).

[17]   Daniel Mornet, *Les Sciences de la nature en France au XVIIIe siècle: Un Chapitre de l'histoire des idées* (Paris: Armand Colin, 1911), 71.

[18]   Among others, Roy Porter proposes that Descartes's *Discourse on Method* (1637) was not primarily an attempt to prove the separate existence of the soul but rather a concerted effort to advance the pursuit of natural science in the face of the Church's proscriptions

century, dualism was well accepted, and the vitalist contestation of its principles would have appeared all the more dangerous in the eyes of Church authorities in that many vitalist medical treatises were written for educated lay persons.

In response to these potential dangers, the vitalists took great care in framing their theories, as Elizabeth A. Williams remarks: "Although Montpellier writings on the vital principle were determinedly secular in tone, never resorting to divine action or intervention to explain the workings of nature or the body, they were also determinedly respectful of orthodoxy, religious feeling, and the church."[19] The vitalists' freedom to gloss over religious questions was guaranteed by more than mere circumspection however, for they were popular with some of the most powerful figures of the era. Anne Vila notes of the materialist connotations of vitalist theories of sensibility: "One factor underlying the greater French tolerance for sensibility's physicalist connotations was the unusual appeal that medicine held for this nation's intellectual and social elite."[20]

The first meaningful attacks on mechanism came from the important vitalist precursor Georg Ernst Stahl, a German chemist and physician who emphasized the role of an active, physiologically invested "soul" in the body's functions.[21] François Boissier de Sauvages de la Croix was the first of the Montpellier Medical School physicians to incorporate Stahl's *anima* into his medical philosophy, an approach that assures him pride of place as the first of the vitalists.[22] Roy Porter concisely summarizes Stahl's influence on vitalist thought: "Organisms were more than the sum of their parts, and purposive human actions could not be explained by mechanical chain reactions alone; activity presupposed the guiding purposive power of a soul. This *anima* was the agent of consciousness and physiological

---

(*Flesh in the Age of Reason: The Modern Foundations of Body and Soul* [New York: Norton, 2003], 65). For Descartes's views on women, see Chapter 5 of Rebecca M. Wilkin's *Women, Imagination, and the Search for Truth in Early Modern France* (Aldershot, UK and Burlington, VT: Ashgate, 2008).

[19]   Williams, *The Physical and the Moral*, 63.

[20]   Anne C. Vila, *Enlightenment and Pathology: Sensibility in the Literature and Medicine of Eighteenth-Century France* (Baltimore: Johns Hopkins University Press, 1998), 3. Other scholarly works on sensibility include R. F. Brissenden, *Virtue in Distress: Studies in the Novel of Sentiment from Richardson to Sade* (New York: Barnes and Noble, 1974); G. J. Barker-Benfield, *The Culture of Sensibility: Sex and Society in Eighteenth-Century Britain* (Chicago: University of Chicago Press, 1992); Janet Todd, *Sensibility: An Introduction* (London: Methuen, 1986); and John C. O'Neal, *The Authority of Experience: Sensationist Theory in the French Enlightenment* (University Park: Pennsylvania State University Press, 1996).

[21]   For a detailed study of Stahl's anima and its decisive effect on the Montpellier school, see Paul Hoffman, "L'Ame et les passions dans la philosophie médicale de Georg-Ernst Stahl," *Dix-Huitième Siècle* 23 (1991): 31–43.

[22]   Sauvages's principal research focus was on women's diseases and the mind–body link. For a discussion of Sauvages on women, see Elizabeth A. Williams, *A Cultural History of Medical Vitalism in Enlightenment Montpellier* (Aldershot, UK and Burlington, VT: Ashgate, 2003), 232–5.

regulation, and disease was the soul's attempt to expel morbid matter and re-establish bodily order."[23] But as Roselyne Rey points out, the vitalists did not embrace the whole of Stahl's doctrines, for his *anima* was similar in its exclusivity to the mechanists' reliance on matter alone: "The Stahlians' use of the soul to explain all physiological or pathological phenomena seemed in the end too symmetrical with the mechanist position, for both were based on the impossibility of thinking of matter as anything other than passive and inert."[24]

Roussel's long panegyric to Stahl in *The Physical and Moral System of Woman* highlights the importance of Stahl's influence: "By making the soul the principle of all our vital movements, [Stahl] overturned the barrier that separated medicine from philosophy. In accordance with his teachings, one can no longer be a doctor without understanding the play of the passions, the influence of habits, and the difference between an active machine whose movements are spontaneous, and a machine moved by a system of inanimate springs."[25] In addition to praising Stahl, Roussel attacks Boerhaave, said to have triumphed only through the machinations of his supporters and his grandiose style, and gives a mixed blessing to Descartes. He elevates above all others Théophile de Bordeu, who was, alongside his sometime rival Paul-Joseph Barthez, the most influential of the early Montpellier vitalists. Bordeu left Montpellier for the greater glory of the French capital, establishing his practice definitively in Paris in 1746. He became known as a specialist in *la médecine galante*, or the curing of the female maladies of Parisian high society. In addition to his many publications, Bordeu contributed one article, "Crisis," to the *Encyclopédie*, but it was among the most famous. His influence on Diderot is most famously evident in *D'Alembert's Dream*, in which Diderot creates a fictionalized version of the well-known doctor.

What most impresses Roussel about Bordeu's work is his well-known theory of "cellular tissue," expounded in *Research on Mucous Tissue, or the Cellular Organ* (1767). "Mucous tissue"—connective tissue, in modern terminology—was so called because it resembled, in Bordeu's terms, a mucilaginous foam (*bave*) or glue (*colle*) that, under a primitive microscope, appeared to be composed of small, almost transparent particles. This tissue was said by Bordeu to fill the body and form cavities for the other organs. By virtue of its expansiveness, this "cellular organ" allowed communication among the body's other organs, with

---

[23]   Roy Porter, *The Greatest Benefit to Mankind: A Medical History of Humanity* (New York: Norton, 1997), 147.

[24]   Roselyne Rey, *Naissance et développement du vitalisme en France de la deuxième moitié du XVIII*e *siècle à la fin du Premier Empire* (Oxford: Voltaire Foundation, 2000), 3. Peter Reill connects the rise of the term "vitalism"—an eighteenth-century neologism, dating to at least 1775 in French—to the need to distinguish the goals of this medical philosophy from those of mechanism and animism (*Vitalizing Nature in the Enlightenment* [Berkeley: University of California Press, 2005], 12).

[25]   Pierre Roussel, *The Physical and Moral System of Woman, or Philosophical Tableau of the Constitution, the Organic State, the Mores, and the Functions Peculiar to the Female Sex* (Paris: Vincent, 1775), xvi–xvii. Roussel's treatise went through seven editions between 1775 and 1869.

the specific density of an individual's mucous tissue considered the key to the quality of this communication, and thus to his or her degree of *sensibilité* (this theory is most evident in Diderot's *Dream* when "Bordeu" compares the living body to a swarm of interconnected bees). Dorinda Outram describes Bordeu's overall influence as follows: "Until Bordeu's work, the 'superior' functions of the body had been attributed to a soul, or to an intellectual or conscious centre, often tacitly considered to be sui generis; but in Bordeu, not only did the soul appear to be cut off from any actual psychic process, but the 'monarchic' supremacy of the conscious intellectual centre is replaced by a federation of many bodily centres."[26]

While prized in general in the eighteenth century as a sign of superiority, the quality of being *sensible*, or of possessing a highly reactive system, was also viewed as a potential cause of illness.[27] Given that female bodies, with their "loose tissue," were said to be particularly subject to such disorders, *sensibilité* is an important aspect of the vitalists' writings on women, but is not the focus of my study. What interests me is above all the variability attributed to sexed differences by the vitalists, and in particular the transformation of unsexed into sexed bodies at puberty, with all the possible perversions and permutations created by an individual's circumstances (including climate) and temperament. Where the treatment of such illness was concerned, the vitalists again emphasized the individual in his or her context, rather than viewing disease, in the manner of the mechanists, as a precise, unchanging point of chemical or mechanical difficulty, easily cured by cutting or by a "specific" remedy (*un spécifique*) designed to purge. As this emphasis on prevention and noninterventionism indicates, the advent of vitalism signaled a profound philosophical reinvention of the physician. In addition to his individual patients, this new type of doctor was viewed as having a duty to the culture at large, including that of educating the growing number of literate lay people.

Another important early figure in the history of vitalism is Bordeu's uncle, Louis de La Caze, who received his medical degree at Montpellier in 1723 and then moved to Paris, as would his nephew after him. La Caze is important to the history of vitalism for his development of the notion of "animal economy," or the interconnectedness of the body's functions, a theory that would be incorporated into Bordeu's essay on connective tissue.[28] La Caze developed "animal economy" in the *Physical and Moral Idea of Man, Intended to Serve as an Introduction to a Treatise on Medicine* (1755), although many of his assumptions are not characteristic of the true vitalists who came later, his nephew included. Rather than stressing the quality of the body's humors, excreted by various organs, La Caze is interested above all in the ingestion of air to the bodily systems.

[26] Dorinda Outram, *The Body and the French Revolution: Sex, Class, and Political Culture* (New Haven: Yale University Press, 1989), 55.

[27] Anne Vila explores the pathology of sensibility in eighteenth-century medical and literary expression in France in *Enlightenment and Pathology* (1998).

[28] For La Caze's relationship to vitalism, see Rey, *Naissance et développement du vitalisme*, 14.

It is air that is said to awaken the body at birth, with the fetus before this moment said to be a mere parasite on its mother. Most notably, while La Caze refers to "the distinctive character of the two sexes," that is, to all the physical and moral differences observable between men and women, these differences are for him of degree and not of kind.[29] The genital fluids that will be so important to later vitalist treatises are not of interest to La Caze; he attributes menstruation in women to the buildup of "phrenic" (diaphragmatic) forces in the uterus.

What will allow the vitalist revolution in sexual differentiation is a combination of the rejection of dualism, La Caze's theory of animal economy, and finally, a revised view of the humors. This last is presented with brevity and clarity in the *Encyclopédie* article "Humor" (no author given), published in 1765. As Elizabeth A. Williams notes, the influence of the vitalists on the presentation of medicine in the *Encyclopédie* increased dramatically after the first volumes appeared. Volumes 8–17 (H–Z), which appeared in a rush in 1765, include the work of a number of Montpellier-trained doctors.[30] "Humor" is in the first of these volumes, and it is heavily marked by vitalism. We are first treated to a summary of the classical vision of the humors as developed in the Hippocratic corpus (fourth century B. C.), according to which temperament was determined by prevailing bodily fluids (*chymoi*). What interests this author, however, is not the elaboration of this ancient system of four humors into its many potential combinations or temperaments, but rather the action of each particular humor upon the organs it influences.

The author accordingly proposes a theory of the humors that will be crucial to vitalist theories of the female body. He declares that the most "natural" division of the humors is into two types: those that serve to aid the conservation of the individual body, and those that serve the propagation of the species. These first are "continually renewed from the instant of conception until death," a necessary continuity in that they nourish the body and thus sustain life. The second of the two "natural" divisions of the humors includes those not present from birth, but rather "produced only at the age at which they may be usefully employed, such as seminal fluid and milk."[31] Whoever wrote this article was far more interested in the second of these "natural" divisions, that is, those humors that appear at prescribed moments in an individual's life and play a critical role in the continuation of the human species. Perhaps the most striking distinction possessed by bodily fluids of this second variety, according to the author of this article, is that they are created for the express purpose of entering another body, be it by impregnating a woman or nursing a child. The health of a child is directly affected by the quality of the sperm his father secretes and the milk produced by his mother's body.

---

[29]   Louis de La Caze, *Idée de l'homme physique et moral, pour servir d'Introduction à un Traité de Médecine* (Paris: Guérin and Delatour, 1755), 280.

[30]   Williams, *A Cultural History*, 120–24. For a complete discussion of the relationship between the vitalists and the Encyclopedists, see Chapter 5 of Williams's study, 147–84.

[31]   *Encyclopédie, ou Dictionnaire raisonné des sciences, des arts et des métiers*, ed. Denis Diderot and Jean d'Alembert (Paris: Briasson [etc.], 1751–1765), VIII:349.

Controlling such variables in the health of young French men and women was the object of the vitalist hygiene treatises. Like the milk ingested by an infant, the cultural influences this growing child would go on to encounter mattered as much as the solid food he or she would eat, the clothing he or she would wear, and the air he or she would breathe. Like La Caze, other early vitalists were known for their work on such classic environmental influences as air and water; Bordeu and other members of his family were known as an experts in the use and promotion of water cures, while Sauvages published an important treatise on the effects of the atmosphere on the human body that begins: "This immense sphere of Air, of which the Earth is the core, is called the *Atmosphere*; Man, as well as the other terrestrial bodies, is immersed in this fluid."[32]

Climate or environmental theory dates back to at least the Hippocratic treatise *On Airs, Waters, and Places* (400 B. C.), and the vitalists could assume a knowledge of the subject in their readers.[33] But while the key environmental influences on health and temperament were traditionally listed as temperature, diet, and mores—in that order—the hygiene theorists of the mid-eighteenth century moved "mores" to the top of this trio of causal agents. The writers of the hygiene treatises on puberty also stand out from previous writers on climate, most notably Montesquieu and Buffon, in that they focus their attacks on degeneracy within their own culture, rather than listing the deleterious effect of environment on such far-flung peoples as the Laps, the Greenlanders, the Africans, and the Americans. I will end this introduction with a brief consideration of the specificity of vitalist environmental theory, as their unique view of the external influences on the human organism is central to the hygiene treatises I go on to consider in the next two chapters.

The *Spirit of the Laws* (1748) by Charles de Secondat, baron de Montesquieu is the best-known work on climate theory written in eighteenth-century France. Jean Ehrard observes that this highly influential work is credited with transforming environmental theory from a relatively simple debate on "national character" into a complex vision that would contribute to the birth of the disciplines of sociology and political science.[34] But while the complexity with which Montesquieu theorizes the relationship between physiology and cultural mores made his writings a central influence on many of the vitalist treatises, the *Spirit of the Laws* possesses none of their prescriptive and proscriptive intensity. The formula of climatic and social phenomena as Montesquieu presents it is self-regulating and tends toward

---

[32] François Boissier de Sauvages de la Croix, *Dissertation où l'on recherche comment l'air, suivant ses différentes qualités, agit sur le corps humain* (Bordeaux: La Veuve de Pierre Brun, 1753), 3.

[33] For the classic history of climate theory, see Clarence J. Glacken, *Traces on the Rhodian Shore: Nature and Culture in Western Thought from Ancient Times to the End of the Eighteenth Century* (Berkeley: University of California Press, 1967).

[34] Jean Ehrard, *L'Idée de nature en France dans la première moitié du XVIIIᵉ siècle*, 2 vols (Paris: S.E.V.P.E.N., 1963), II:719.

equilibrium. The closest he comes to criticizing French women is his reference to the self-serving machinations of the noble women who frequent Versailles, but again, this influence is presented as a necessary outgrowth of the monarchical form of government. The character of French women is as much a product of the temperate French climate as is the French government. Even the age of onset of menses in French women is said to be climate dependent and yet another cause of the relative social freedom they enjoy as behind-the-scenes political forces. Montesquieu notes that in Oriental societies, heat-induced early puberty leads men to marry girls who are still mentally children, with the result that Oriental women never establish adult relationships with their husbands and are accorded none of the relative freedom enjoyed by European women (see Book XVI of the *Spirit of the Laws*, "On how the laws of domestic slavery are in accord with the nature of climate"). But again, Montesquieu is not pointing to such "evidence" in order to denounce polygamy and seraglios; he is merely making a statement of fact to which he attaches little to no moral judgment.

George-Louis Leclerc, comte de Buffon, was another important influence in renewing interest in the effects of climate theory on human societies in the mid-eighteenth century. He addresses the topic in "Varieties of the Human Species," the third volume of his *Natural History* (1749). Buffon is far more detailed in his analysis of the supposed influences of climate than is Montesquieu, giving the reader a long list of racial distinctions cited from an impressive number of travel narratives, with each tied to specific latitudes. We read, for example: "The most temperate climate is that between the 40th and 50th degrees, and one therefore finds in this zone the best-looking men" (III:528). This citation illustrates an important commonality in the use of environmental theory by Buffon and Montesquieu: the presence in their works of a discourse in which a racist sense of one's own cultural superiority happily coexists with the assumption of scientific objectivity. For the vitalists, the complacent assumption that the temperate climate was indeed ideal for the development of human civilization was undone by the belief that this very suitability had led the Europeans to cross the line, to divert too far from the natural path and thus to fall victim to an ever-accelerating process of degradation. The apocalyptical opening of Jean-Jacques Rousseau's *Emile, ou de l'éducation* (1761) is only slightly more hyperbolic than the viewpoint of the average vitalist: "Everything degenerates in the hands of man ... he overturns everything, he disfigures everything, he loves deformities, monsters; he wants nothing as nature made it, not even man ... Quickly erect a fence around the soul of your child."[35]

Buffon's relationship with vitalism has been explored by a number of historians of science, given that he is both a distinct precursor and in some ways a sympathetic contemporary to vitalism. Roselyne Rey notes that Buffon's professional career overlaps the first wave of vitalist writings, and that he served as something of a mediator for the vitalists by means of his "reinterpretation of Newtonianism

---

[35]   Jean-Jacques Rousseau, *Emile, ou de l'éducation*, in *Oeuvres complètes*, 4 vols (Paris: Gallimard, 1959–1969), IV:245–6.

and his rereading of Leibnitz."[36] But although Buffon stressed the existence of a "life principle" and was an antimechanist in his insistence on the radical duality of life and death, his Cartesianism separated him from the vitalist school in a significant manner.[37] Part of the problem is the mutability of the term "vitalism," a movement that can best be termed a "current" of thought, for the vitalists were a heterogeneous group in many respects.

Optimism about the future of the human race should be added to Rey's list of distinctions between Buffonism and vitalism. The famous Buffonian *moule intérieur*, or "inner mold," to which each species must remain faithful, even as it is modified by the forces of climate and multiplication, includes in the case of humans the instinct to reach as high a degree of civilization as possible.[38] The rewards for this effort are clear, for Buffon: "A civilized people, living with a certain ease, accustomed to a regulated existence, sweet and tranquil, who are protected from extreme poverty by a good government ... will be composed of stronger, better-looking, and better-made men that those of a savage and independent nation" (IV:446–7). Emma Spary notes that while this "civilized" state is precarious and carries no guarantee of continuation, Buffon nevertheless celebrates the perfectible mind of man: "Buffon's nature was ... constantly degenerating, falling into gradual decay and ultimate death. In the *Histoire naturelle*, Buffon offset this negative trend with man's ingenuity and ability to combat degeneration through the advancements that the sciences, the arts, and society could bring."[39]

In the treatises that I consider, Europeans have no one to blame for their sad state and imminent destruction but themselves, and advancement in the sciences is not the answer except insofar as it enables us to return to nature's precepts. Take for example the "Preliminary Discourse" to the *Treatise on the Corporal Education of Young Children* (1760) by Jean-Charles Desessartz, a work said to have strongly influenced Jean-Jacques Rousseau's portrayal of puberty in *Emile*. A prominent Parisian doctor, Desessartz addresses his and his culture's growing concern about depopulation by proposing a solution based on improved hygiene (his subtitle is "Practical Reflections on How to Improve the Constitution of Citizens").[40] He has little sympathy for those who blame nature for this decline, declaring them to be

---

[36]   Roselyne Ray, "Buffon et le vitalisme" in *Buffon 88: actes du Colloque international pour le bicentenaire de la mort de Buffon* (Paris: J. Vrin, 1992), 400.

[37]   Rey, "Buffon et le vitalisme," 399–400. Peter Reill views Buffon's most important contribution in this context to be that he "broke the spell" of systems; for Reill, the first three volumes of the *Histoire naturelle* constitute the symbolic starting point for the coming, widespread "new language" of nature (*Vitalizing Nature*, 31).

[38]   For an analysis of the philosophical basis for the Buffonian *moule intérieur*, see Reill, *Vitalizing Nature*, 47.

[39]   Emma Spary, *Utopia's Garden: French Natural History from Old Regime to Revolution* (Chicago: University of Chicago Press, 2000), 32.

[40]   For more on the belief that the population of Europe was declining, see Carol Blum, *Strength in Numbers: Population, Reproduction, and Power in Eighteenth-Century France* (Baltimore: Johns Hopkins University Press, 2002).

hiding behind "a miserable pretext born of pride and used to disguise the vices of our moral conduct and all that we do, the true cause of the disappearance of the human species."[41] That climate has nothing to do with the current disaster faced by urban Europeans is clear when he points to the Savoy and the Auvergne as locations so populous that they must export many inhabitants each year to Paris, and declares that the reason for this healthy output of children is that "sobriety and work" are the norm in these areas.

Louis de Lignac also insists that we must not blame nature for our self-induced problems.[42] Lignac is not averse to climate theory, and even cites a 1760 report by one M. Pibrac, who studied the effects of what one might call "microclimates." Pibrac believed that the effects of "climate" were evident on the level of individual Parisian neighborhoods, even streets, and claimed that the strongest men and therefore those best suited for militia duty came from the Faubourgs St. Martin and St. Denis.[43] But despite citing with apparent approbation this extreme form of environmental determinism, Lignac begins his treatise, as did Desessartz, with a strong statement concerning the moral causes of the degeneration he sees all around him. We are at fault, he insists, not nature; we are sexualized too early, we marry the wrong types of partners, and as a result, we produce weak offspring who go on to do the same.[44]

Writers such as Lignac represent a mid-point between Montesquieu and Buffon's satisfaction with the superiority of their cultural status quo and the coming Revolutionary fervor for the "new man." The optimism of this last generation in the face of a degradation they still accepted as truth is epitomized by a statement in the *Sketch of an Historical Tableau of the Progress of the Human Mind* (1795) by Jean-Antoine-Nicolas de Caritat, marquis de Condorcet. At the end of the "Second Epoch" of his ten-part *Sketch*, Condorcet ponders why positive social developments such as the domestication of animals and agriculture are not accompanied by a correspondingly positive development in human virtue and happiness. He notes that the contrary seems to be at times the case, but he

---

[41]   Jean-Charles Desessartz, *Traité de l'éducation corporelle des enfants en bas âge ou Réflexions pratiques sur les moyens de procurer une meilleure constitution aux citoyens* (Paris: Herissant, 1760), ix–x.

[42]   Little is known about Louis de Lignac other than that he was a surgeon, as is declared on the title page of his treatise, *De l'Homme et de la femme considérés physiquement dans l'état de mariage* (1772), a work that, despite the current obscurity of its author, quickly went through several French editions in the 1770s (it appeared in German in 1772; in Italian in 1785; in Swedish in 1797; in English in 1798). He is not to be confused with the materialist philosopher Joseph Adrien Lelarge de Lignac, enemy of Buffon and author of *Lettres à un Amériquain* (1751).

[43]   Lignac writes that M. Pibrac read this report in 1760 before the Académie Royale de Chirurgerie (*De l'Homme et de la femme considérés physiquement dans l'état de mariage*, 2 vols [Lille: J. B. Henry, 1772], II:125–6). Lignac's work is much informed by the *Tableau de l'amour conjugal* of Nicolas Venette, first published in Amsterdam in 1675.

[44]   Lignac, *De l'Homme et de la femme*, I:2–3.

then insists nonetheless on the ongoing, continual evidence of the perfectibility of the human race. Enlightenment is always a force for good, we are told, for at the very least it softens those human vices it cannot eliminate: "So we will see that the stormy and painful passage from a rough, unformed society to the civilized state of enlightened and free peoples is not at all a degeneration of the human species, but rather a crisis that is necessary to its gradual progress toward absolute perfection."[45]

In contrast, the physiologists influenced by vitalist thought were far from confident in the future. Roselyne Rey summarizes the despair at the heart of the vitalist writings: "More than any other current [of medical philosophy], vitalism expressed a frustration with the gulf between confidence in the perfectibility of the human mind, the conviction that a new era is about to dawn, and the few results achieved."[46] For Lignac, we are almost no better than the "Samoyeds," who live in an ice-cold climate but whose young children nevertheless experience early puberty as a consequence of their huddling for most of the year in crowded cabins, where they are regularly exposed to sexual activity. The result is said to be such a deformed adult population that one can scarcely distinguish between the Samoyed men and women.[47] According to the treatises that proliferated in France beginning in the 1760s, the dangers inherent in French culture, in the rather less dramatic form of novels, were as destructive as the promiscuous Samoyed lifestyle, and above all to young girls. The resulting obsession with a secular moral purity of the most negative sort—passive, born of protection from cultural influences deemed decadent, and lasting until a young girl's wedding night—would have significant repercussions for the cultural configuration of ideal womanhood for some time to come.

Sean Quinlan notes of the movement toward government intervention in matters of health that took place from 1750 to 1850 that the ultimate goal was to create a blueprint for a better society:

> Medical practitioners thus explored problems that we do not always associate with public health: ideal health and beauty; how men and women should behave and what roles they should play in public and private life; how parents should raise and teach their children, and how to improve sexual hygiene and fertility. At times, physicians focused upon real or imagined behaviour in particular groups of people, and they changed their objects of study and approbation as the political and social context changed over the age of revolution.[48]

---

[45]   Jean-Antoine-Nicolas de Caritat, marquis de Condorcet, *Esquisse d'un tableau historique des progrès de l'esprit humain* (Paris: Vrin, 1970), 58.

[46]   Rey, *Naissance et développement du vitalisme*, 15.

[47]   Lignac, *De l'Homme et de la femme*, II:241–2.

[48]   Sean M. Quinlan, *The Great Nation in Decline: Sex, Modernity and Health Crises in Revolutionary France c. 1750–1850* (Aldershot, UK and Burlington, VT: Ashgate, 2007), 5.

While the object of concern did indeed change over the 100-year period that concerns Quinlan, I would argue that the ingénue was the original and remained a key cause of medical concern in that she embodied, as the mid-century physiologists conceived her, the central problematic at the heart of the Enlightenment: the pull between the benefits of nature and those of culture. The complex discourse on civilization and nature epitomized by the ingénue is the central cautionary tale of the Enlightenment project at a whole, one common to physiological, fictional, and ultimately, political discourse.

Chapter 1
Puberty and the Splitting of the Single Sex

[Puberty] is a true fermentation that necessarily produces a new being. Yes, Nature, occupied with her masterpiece, is like a mother giving birth. She suffers fears, agitations, and pains that must be stimulated when they are slow or false, and moderated when they come too quickly or last too long.
—Guillaume Daignan, *Tableau of the Varieties of Human Life* (1786)

Historians and cultural theorists have argued that the eighteenth century witnessed the solidification of such diverse cultural phenomena as the public sphere, pornography, and the modern self.[1] One of the most influential and certainly the most provocative of such claims comes from Thomas Laqueur: "Sometime in the eighteenth century, sex as we know it was invented."[2] Laqueur is not referring of course to the sex act in all its diversity, but rather to the rejection of the isomorphic vision of sexual difference that held the female to be an inversion of the normative male. This Galenic tenet was made possible by the gross structural similarities between the ovaries and the testicles on the one hand and the uterus and the penis on the other. The resulting theory viewed women as so many "men" whose colder, earthlike qualities had not allowed the descent of their virile parts. As Laqueur argues, the eighteenth century witnessed the replacement of this vision of relative sameness by the two-sex model, a physiological theory that held men and women to be qualitatively distinct.

In elaborating on Laqueur's insight, historians of medicine have argued that this ideological rupture should not be primarily attributed to seventeenth- and eighteenth-century discoveries concerning the configuration of the human female genital organs.[3] Michael Stolberg, for example, has shown that anatomical works from the sixteenth century demonstrate a clear understanding of the male and

---

[1]   On the public sphere, see Jürgen Habermas, *The Structural Transformation of the Public Sphere* (in German, 1962; first English translation 1989); on pornography, Robert Darnton, *The Forbidden Best-Sellers of Pre-Revolutionary France* (1996); on the modern self, Charles Taylor, *Sources of the Self* (1989).

[2]   Thomas W. Laqueur, *Making Sex: Body and Gender from the Greeks to Freud* (Cambridge, MA: Harvard University Press, 1990), 149.

[3]   See for example Peter Hanns Reill, *Vitalizing Nature in the Enlightenment* (Berkeley: University of California Press, 2005), 222. The most complete treatment of this subject is Elizabeth A. Williams's *A Cultural History of Medical Vitalism in Enlightenment Montpellier* (Aldershot, UK and Burlington, VT: Ashgate, 2003), along with her earlier *The Physical and the Moral: Anthropology, Physiology, and Philosophical Medicine in France, 1750–1850* (Cambridge: Cambridge University Press, 1994). Williams cites Foucault's *The Birth of the Clinic* (1963) as the beginning of the revival of interest in Montpellier vitalism.

female genitalia as distinct.[4] The "invention" of sex involved, to the contrary, the rejection of such structural concerns, and was in great part the result of the revival by the Montpellier vitalists of a different aspect of Galenic physiology: humoralism. The vitalists revised humoral theory to suit their fascination with sexual difference, arguing that rather than two versions of the same fluid, the male and female genital humors were absolutely distinct in nature and, just as significantly, were the most dramatically transformative of the body's vital forces.

Women had always of course been considered a "separate" sex, but this new vision of women replaced two extremes of the same model with two distinct models, leading the physiologists to marvel that men and women belonged to the same species. To borrow a term from Londa Schiebinger, this ideological rupture constitutes a "resexualization" of the body.[5] The eighteenth-century physiologists of puberty were not at all interested in the structure of the penis, the vagina, the clitoris, or the breasts, but rather in the genital fluids understood as animating essences. The clearest expression of this lack of concern with the structure of the genitalia is also the topic of the present chapter: the insistence in the eighteenth-century treatises on puberty that boy and girl children are "identical" until they begin the transformative process of puberty. "Identical" is meant to convey that the genital organs of these mucous filled, unfinished, unreasoning creatures are not yet actively pumping out their own, unique type of fluid. In the terminology of the hygiene treatises, the genitals are "asleep" throughout the years of childhood growth and "awaken" only at puberty, when they begin to produce these humors and release them into the bloodstream, utterly transforming the child's body and mind.

Daignan's *Tableau of the Varieties of Human Life* (1786) is a relatively late entry into this corpus of treatises and of great value for this reason, for he brings together the principal assumptions of previous authors whose works focused on the hygiene of puberty. The title page of Daignan's treatise identifies him as a Montpellier doctor, and the work's full, lengthy title indeed reads as something of a manifesto for the vitalist view of puberty: *Tableau of the Varieties of Human Life, with the advantages and disadvantages of each constitution and some very important advice for fathers and mothers considering the health of their children, of both sexes, especially at the age of puberty; in which we demonstrate, that at this time, most sicknesses must not be considered as such, but rather as the salutary efforts of nature to develop the organs; and that serious illnesses must be treated with more care and circumspection, than at any other age.*

The precise connotations of the word "variety" as Daignan uses it reveal his Montpellier training as much as the proud declaration of place found on his title page. By "varieties of human life," we are to understand above all not the "racial" differences in the human species that so obsessed the era's natural historians, but

---

    [4]   Michael Stolberg, "A Woman Down to Her Bones," *Isis* 94 (2003): 274–99. Londa Schiebinger also explores this question in Chapters 7 and 8 of *The Mind Has No Sex? Women in the Origins of Modern Science* (Cambridge, MA: Harvard University Press, 1989).

    [5]   Londa Schiebinger, *The Mind Has No Sex?* 190.

rather individual differences in temperament among French children. Parents are to learn in the work that only an understanding of their child's specific humoral configuration will allow them to manipulate his or her innate constitution in order to produce a fixed, healthy adult temperament. The influence of climate on national characteristics still plays a role for Daignan, but because airs, waters, and places act on such a large scale, environmental theory is of far less importance to his physiological approach than it was for Buffon or Montesquieu.

The didacticism with which Daignan addresses his readers in his title, telling them what they "must" and "must not" do, reflects the acceptance of this social role for doctors by 1786. The institutionalization of the vitalist hygiene theories was well underway by this date, most notably via the founding of the Royal Society of Medicine with funds allotted by Louis XVI, and with the mandate to improve public health.[6] Daignan's focus on teaching the public about this particular period of human development reflects another significant cultural change occurring in the mid-eighteenth century as well: the "invention" of adolescence. While the word *adolescence* dates in French to the end of the thirteenth century, the belief that this period between childhood and adulthood merited particular attention and its own theoretical development was certainly new.[7] Daignan's title indicates that only by buying and studying his treatise will parents be enlightened as to how to handle behaviors and physical issues in their pubescent (adolescent) children that they might otherwise not even have noticed, so unaccustomed are they to considering this period as an important developmental stage. The reference to the "serious illnesses" that accompany this passage to adulthood is clearly meant to frighten potential readers, who are to accede to Daignan's medical expertise or risk confusing a problem in need of a cure with one of the "salutary" effects of nature that mimic illness and are to be left alone to work their transformative magic.

Adolescence has perhaps never since been portrayed as such a difficult, dangerous, and yet ultimately exhilarating time for both children and their parents than when it first appeared as a medical and social phenomenon in the eighteenth century. This excessive concern is in great part the product of the instability attributed by the vitalists to human existence in general, at all periods of life. Prepubescent children are also said to be in constant danger from disease due to their loose, mucousy state, and adults are relatively unstable despite their fixed temperament, for the genital fluids are said to be continually produced and reabsorbed into the bloodstream throughout adulthood. These unsettling effects disappear only when menarche

---

[6] See Sean M. Quinlan, *The Great Nation in Decline: Sex, Modernity and Health Crises in Revolutionary France c. 1750–1850* (Aldershot, UK and Burlington, VT: Ashgate, 2007), 53. Daignan's role in this institutionalization is evident as well in his *Military Gymnastics* (1790) in which, as a "consultant" to the King's armies, he details the hygiene regime best suited to produce "strong and robust" soldiers.

[7] The *Dictionnaire de l'Académie française* specifies until at least the 6th edition of 1835 that the noun and adjective forms (*adolescence, adolescent*) are used only for boys; but Diderot refers to "adolescent boys and girls" in his *Supplément au voyage de Bougainville*, in *Oeuvres* (Paris: Gallimard, 1951), 983.

occurs, we learn, although we are not to greet this stability with delight. Menarche is defined as the point when the genitals cease producing their sexed humors and men and women return once again to a (physically and mentally deflated) state of "identity," the precursor to the slow devitalization that ends in death.

As the disappearance of sex difference in this last stage of life demonstrates, sexuation is to be understood as neither a fixed nor a permanent phenomenon in the works I am examining. According to the two-sex model as the vitalists present it, maleness and femaleness are temporary and fluctuating states. Our standard cultural notions of sex difference as both signified by the outward form of the genitalia (whatever variations may occur) and embedded in the most profound (genetic) structures of the body, must be discarded in approaching works in which sex characteristics, like any other aspect of temperament, come and go in intensity and at times even in essence.

In the first part of this chapter, I detail how the creation and flow of the sexed genital fluids at puberty is said to "give birth" to the two sexes. In the second part, I consider the dangers associated with this passage from childhood to young adulthood, and most importantly the potential mental disturbances attributed to young people at this time, some salutary, some indicative of disease. By far the most dangerous of these mental manifestations of puberty is said to be the intense feelings of physical desire awakened when the genitals are first simulated by the action of their rich humors. Parents are told that they must at all costs prevent their children from recognizing the sexual nature of these sensations and thereby realizing that sexual activity, masturbatory or otherwise, relieves such stimulating, uncomfortable sensations. While the need to protect girls from knowledge is emphasized over the protection of boys, the latter are said to have far more to lose in the mental realm by the premature spilling of their *liqueur*. The relatively neglected female humor is said to possess little of the "fortifying" and "vivifying" qualities attributed to "male" semen, a sex difference that condemns even healthy, "innocent" young women to something like an eternal childhood. The ingénue will soon be "injected" with this male fluid however, on her wedding night, and my rather lengthy discussion of "male" semen in the last part of this chapter is intended to prepare the exploration of this key transformative event in women's lives in the following chapter.

Vitalism, Variability, and the Two-Sex Model

The medical historian Elizabeth A. Williams emphasizes the centrality of variability to the vitalist philosophy of medicine:

> [The] acceptance, indeed valorization, of the variability of "life-phenomena" encouraged Montpellier theorists to take up problems surrounding growth and aging that were necessarily slighted in mechanist analyses of body function. If the body was in fact a clocklike machine as Descartes had insisted, its slow and subtle transformations throughout life were difficult to explain. Vitalist medicine gave special attention to growth and aging, tracing for each of the four "stages

of life" (childhood, youth, maturity, old age) the relative proportions and "influence" of the peculiar conditions and diseases characteristic of that stage.[8]

While childhood, youth, maturity, and old age occupy some space in the treatises I consider in this chapter, the passage from childhood to youth, understood as the intense explosion of intellectual and physical development that occurs at puberty, receives by far the most attention. The hygiene of puberty is presented as a central public health concern, given the young person's potential to deviate from nature's prescribed path. Fears about the negative cultural effects of any such deviation, on a wide scale, both justified and ensured the publication of how-to handbooks for parents such as Daignan's.

The majority of the hygiene treatises on puberty I consider appeared during the 1760s and 1770s, the decades identified by Williams as marking the turn from the metaphysical to the practical in vitalist discourse. It follows that the earliest and some of the most famous figures of Montpellier vitalism, including Théophile de Bordeu, did not write the type of propagandistic work that interests me in this chapter. Nor are some of the authors whose works I will be citing directly associated with the Montpellier School of Medicine, although the influence of this dominant school upon their writings is strong and includes the choice to write for a general public, rather than an exclusively medical audience. The belief that the systematic application of hygiene theory was the best approach to improving a declining population steeped in unhealthy practices gave to sexual differentiation as the vitalists imagined it a cultural resonance not present in previous medical discussions of the topic. In addition, it generated a rhetoric of near hysteria in some of these treatises, and gave to all of these works a compelling air of immediacy.

The first of what would become a wave of didactic works aimed at changing the hygiene practices of the general public was also among the most strident: Samuel Auguste Tissot's *Onanism* (1760). As Michel Foucault acerbically observed in a lecture at the Collège de France: "Soon after the publication of Tissot's book in France, the problem, the discourse, the immense jabbering about masturbation starts up and does not stop for a whole century."[9] Although Tissot studied medicine at Montpellier before returning to his native Switzerland to practice, he was eclectic in his approach, and the focus on variability and transformation that marks the vitalist works is generally absent from his writings. He did however spend his career admonishing Europeans that they were to change their hygiene practices or face the (drastic) consequences, and many of his meliorist concerns echo those of the vitalists.[10]

---

[8]   Williams, *The Physical and the Moral*, 53.

[9]   Michel Foucault, *Abnormal: Lectures at the Collège de France 1974–1975* (London: Verso, 2003), 233. Sean M. Quinlan sums up the essence of Tissot's writings: "he wanted to reform the bawdy and cheeky world of the mid-Enlightenment, with its sly mix of eroticism, materialism, and philosophic skepticism" (*The Great Nation in Decline*, 39).

[10]   Tissot attacked those who refrained from physical activity (sexual or otherwise) in his *Essay on Men of Letters* (1768) and targeted the worldly elite in his *Essay on the Disorders of People of Fashion* (1770).

The turn to a lay audience by authors who, like Tissot, wrote on matters of sexual hygiene was not without its difficulties. The greatest fear, at least as expressed in these treatises, was that adolescents might be damaged by reading the very treatises intended to help their parents protect them.[11] The descriptive nature of such works was the source of the problem, for in order to prescribe a proper hygienic regime, the authors had to depict exact symptoms and behaviors. Dorinda Outram notes of the vogue for similar works devoted to the care of infants and children at this time: "Previous eras had seen the writing of many books of parental advice to children, and guides to manners and morals composed for them. But the family of the late eighteenth century was the first to compile manuals of actual care of the infant and small child which went into minute detail about the direction of its physical existence."[12] Once this child—in whom, it was assumed, all sexual feeling was absent—began to go through puberty, the "minute details" of its physical life became quite a bit more scandalous and therefore dangerous, as much to the authors as to the supposedly vulnerable adolescent readers.

Buffon was another important nonvitalist influence on the popularization of scientific writings in the eighteenth century. He is said to have had nonspecialists read his works aloud, and to have revised any sections that these readers had trouble understanding.[13] Such efforts paid off in sales and popularity, for as Emma Spary notes, the *Natural History* was "the third most commonly owned work [in the eighteenth century], despite its length and undoubted expense."[14] While Buffon was far more concerned with offending Church authorities with his theories than with arousing adolescent desires, in the portion of his *Natural History* devoted to "The Natural History of Man" he begins his discussion of puberty with a question, followed by an assurance:

> Will we be able to trace the history of this age with enough circumspection to awaken only philosophical ideas in the reader's imagination? Puberty, its accompanying circumstances, circumcision, castration, virginity, impotence, all are so essential to the history of man that we cannot leave out the facts related to them; we will therefore try to enter into such details ... with the

---

[11]   Alexandre Wenger considers the rhetoric of eighteenth-century medical prefaces in *La Fibre littéraire: Le Discours médical sur la lecture au XVIIIᵉ siècle* (Geneva: Droz, 2007), 231–7. As Tissot explains in his preface, *Onanism* was a translation (to which additional material was added) of his essay in Latin on masturbation, *Tentamen de morbis ex manu stupratione*, part of his *Dissertatio de febribus biliosis* (Lausanne, 1758).

[12]   Dorinda Outram, *The Body and the French Revolution: Sex, Class and Political Culture* (New Haven: Yale University Press, 1989), 142.

[13]   J. M. Tanner, *A History of the Study of Human Growth* (Cambridge: Cambridge University Press, 1981), 80.

[14]   Emma Spary, *Utopia's Garden: French Natural History from Old Regime to Revolution* (Chicago: University of Chicago Press, 2000), 26.

philosophical difference that destroys all expressive feeling, and allows words to retain only their most basic meanings.[15]

In the *Treatise on the Maladies of Women* (1761–1765), a book entirely devoted to these "accompanying circumstances," the vitalist Jean Astruc insists that there is one subject simply too obscene to lend itself to the careful euphemisms he employs elsewhere in his study: the wild sexual urges experience by women in the grip of "uterine furors." Astruc was of the early generation of vitalists—he studied and taught in Montpellier before moving to Paris in 1746—and it was in part due to his influence that the work of the second generation of vitalist theoreticians would be marked by an attention to women's illnesses. But while this younger generation will feel free to discuss "uterine furors" and its violent disorders in French, Astruc does not:

> The wish to be useful has caused me to give this treatise in French, so that everyone will be able to read it. I have been troubled by this decision, when required to speak about certain subjects, but I have taken care not to use expressions capable of causing the least shock. This method did not work with regard to *Uterine Furors*. The obscenities at the heart of this illness, which I could not avoid treating, obliged me to write this chapter in Latin.[16]

Efforts to avoid graphic detail include Jean Goulin's statement that in the interest of both modesty and clarity he has attempted as much as possible "to compare this or that part of the human body with the same part of a domesticated animal" (*The Woman's Doctor, or the Art of Keeping Them Healthy*, 1771).[17] In a work published in the same year, *On Nymphomania, or Treatise on Uterine Furors*, J. D. T. de Bienville instead sees the cure in the poison, stating that he has chosen the vernacular precisely in the hope of inspiring horror in nonspecialist readers. Should the book fall into the hands of a young girl, either through parental inattention or through libertine machinations, Bienville assures us that his vivid descriptions of the dangers associated with precocious sexuality will instill horror in her.[18]

---

[15] George-Louis Leclerc, comte de Buffon, *Histoire naturelle, générale et particulière*, 36 vols (Paris: Imprimerie Royale, 1749–1788), II:479. For Buffon's attitude toward religion and struggles with Church censors, see Daniel Mornet, *Les Sciences de la nature en France, au XVIIIe siècle* (Paris: Armand Colin, 1911), 50–71.

[16] Jean Astruc, *Traité des Maladies des femmes*, 6 vols (Paris: Cavelier, 1761–1765), I:xxii.

[17] Jean Goulin, *Le Médecin des dames, ou l'Art de les conserver en santé* (Paris: Vincent, 1771), v. Future references in the text. Little is known of Goulin, despite his many publications; it is not clear where he earned his degree, for example, although it is known that he was forced to stop studying in Paris due to financial reasons.

[18] J. D. T. Bienville, *De La Nymphomanie ou Traité de la fureur utérine* (Amsterdam: Marc-Michel Rey, 1771), ix. Future references in the text. *De La Nymphomanie* went through a number of French editions and was quickly translated into German and English as well; this popularity makes it all the more curious that so little is known of Bienville's life, other than that he may have received a medical degree in Holland.

While "not daring to condemn the excess of modesty in such a respectable man" as Astruc, he laments that no author, ancient or modern, has been willing to treat the topic of uterine furors openly (vi). Consider the incalculable good accomplished by Tissot's "energetic treatise on *Onanism*," we are told, in which "true and frightening images" are painted to great effect (vii). Bienville's concern for his lay readers extends to including an appendix containing precise medicinal formulas for the mixing of medications; he also explains, at the end of his introduction, how to measure precisely such quantities as a pinch, a handful, and a spoonful.

Judging by the popularity of *On Nymphomania*, Bienville succeeded in his goal of reaching his intended readers: those parents possessed of the money and the time to purchase and read such treatises and, presumably, put his prescriptions into effect. There are two stages to these parents' task of shepherding their children to maturity, with the first consisting of guiding one's charge safely through the transformational "crisis" of puberty, universally described in a manner sure to inspire parental concern. Consider, again, Daignan's exemplary *Tableau of the Varieties of Human Life*, in the introduction to which he summarizes the qualities of the pubescent body and mind:

> Everything is at that time lively, sensitive, active, supple, and easily stimulated; all the humors are in a state of effervescence: all the types of vessels are in motion, excited, tickled, bothered, by a redoubled friction, and by the rapid movement of the liquids, they contract, they clench, they stiffen, and produce at times extraordinary effects, which often give rise to irrational fears.[19]

He counsels parents not to be frightened by sudden personality changes, nor even by a sudden, striking physical change, as in the color of a young person's hair or eyes. One sees every day, Daignan comments, "beautiful young blonds who, at this period, become brown-haired, chestnut hair become black, the thin become fat, the weak, strong, the sanguine, phlegmatic, the bilious become melancholic" (I:222).

Once parents have successfully overseen their child's development into a healthy postpubescent—a young adult characterized by a fixed temperament (and presumably stable eye and hair color)—they face a second, only somewhat less arduous task: finding their offspring a suitable mate and timing the marriage correctly. "Marriage" is to be understood as a useful euphemism for "sex," that all-important physical activity the careful management of which is central to any individual's health. Only sexual congress—understood as heterosexual intercourse undertaken with the aim of producing healthy children—will, when the time is right, finally "settle" the still volatile postpubescent body.

Before such advanced worries are to occupy the minds of parents, however, they must deal with those amorphous, nonsexual beings known in these treatises as "children." The "identity" of prepubescent boys and girls was based on their shared state of extreme fluidity and the resulting lack of structure and tension in

---

[19]   Guillaume Daignan, *Tableau des variétés de la vie humaine*, 2 vols (Paris: chez l'Auteur, 1786), I:xiv. Future references in the text.

their bodies and minds. Roussel is unusual in declaring that there may indeed be "a primitive difference" between male and female bodies, but this statement is an aside in his introduction.[20] When he again speculates along these lines, in a note to the main text, it is to hypothesize that differences in male and female bone structure could well be primordial (present at birth), but they might also be due to the penetration of sexed cellular tissue into the bones during and after puberty. He will, he declares, leave the question to the anatomists to decide. By pursuing their structural agendas through autopsies, in other words, the anatomists will discover "the point at which a woman ceases to be a woman, and begins to be a man" (19–20, note). Roussel himself is interested in the far more fascinating, important, and pervasive differences between the sexes.

The ubiquity of the view that young girls and boys were identical in the physical and the moral realms is perhaps best demonstrated by its presence in the famously reductionist treatment of sexual difference in Rousseau's *Emile, or On Education* (1762). When the tutor begins his discussion of Emile's passage to manhood in the opening paragraphs of Book Four, he makes a striking statement concerning the prepuberty equivalence of boys and girls: "Until the age of nubility, children of both sexes have no apparent distinguishing features; the same face, the same figure, the same complexion, the same voice, all is equal; girls are children, boys are children; the same name suffices for such similar beings."[21] This absolute equality is of course to be understood as a (commonly accepted) shared blankness, born of lack of development, but its presence in *Emile* is nevertheless striking. Rousseau also employs the common metaphor of the birth process for puberty, for the tutor informs his readers that we are born in two steps, "one for the species and the other for sex" (489).

The physiology of puberty is indeed fundamental to Rousseau's innovative approach to education, an aspect of this work that has all too often been overlooked.[22] The tutor repeats the second-birth metaphor when he explains that Emile's education, properly understood, can begin only after puberty: "This is the second birth of which I spoke; it is at this point that man is truly born to life and that nothing human is foreign to him ... This epoch, at which ordinary educations finish, is where our own is to begin" (490). The allusion to the Terentian *homo sum* (I am a human being, so nothing human is foreign to me) goes so far as to place the species of prepubescent children into question. If to be human is to have a mind developed enough by the forces of puberty to interest itself in

---

[20] Pierre Roussel, *Système physique et moral de la femme* (Paris: Vincent, 1775), xxviii. Future references in the text.

[21] Jean-Jacques Rousseau, *Emile, ou de l'éducation*, in *Oeuvres complètes*, 4 vols (Paris: Gallimard, 1959–1969), IV:493. Future references in the text.

[22] Gilbert Py notes that like Buffon, Rousseau was often quoted as an expert in eighteenth-century treatises on childhood physiology (*Rousseau et les éducateurs:Etude sur la fortune des idées pédagogiques de Jean-Jacques Rousseau en France et en Europe au XVIIIe siècle* [Oxford: Voltaire Foundation, 1997], 284).

others, and to recognize oneself as a rational being, it follows that to be human is to be postpubescent. Like the authors of the more properly medical hygiene treatises, Rousseau bases his system of negative education on the premise that the prepubescent child is a prerational being. Until puberty has erupted within him, we understand, only direct experience will imprint itself upon Emile's unfixed, malleable brain.[23]

The reader might well get the impression that the treatment of childhood education in *Emile* is merely a preamble to the "birth" of the tutor's charge to full humanity, were it not that this particular preamble covers three-fifths of the entire work. The education proper to Emile's prepubescent years is covered in Books One to Three, with the tutor turning only in Book Four to the question of how any right-thinking guardian must shepherd his male charge through the dangers of puberty. By the end of this book, with maturity looming, Emile is said to be in immediate need of "marriage" to a wife who will, in her fully developed female attributes, complement his carefully nurtured maleness. The education of this ideal woman—a young woman selected by the tutor, of course—is the subject of the fifth and last book, "Sophie, or On Woman." The proper method by which to raise Emile's intended requires a separate chapter because, as readers have (at times angrily) noted since the work's first publication, girls are not to be given the nonprescriptive "negative" education granted to Emile. The role of Sophie's mother—and it is made clear that a girl must be educated by her mother—is to cajole or trick her daughter into sitting quietly and sewing, thereby learning patience and the art of self-suppression.

Liselotte Steinbrügge aptly describes the goal of Sophie's preadolescent training: "All those qualities usually considered feminine, such as a fondness for finery, curiosity, coquetry, adroitness, and garrulousness, which Rousseau describes as 'natural inclinations,' must be channeled in order to prevent excess."[24] In the process Rousseau contradicts his previous assertion that boys and girls are identical, for he alleges, as Steinbrügge notes, that girl children possess an innate interest in dolls and self-adornment. In instructing mothers in how to use this penchant to direct their young daughters' admirable energy toward stillness, however, Rousseau is elaborating an education for girls that is in its basic approach "identical" to that given to Emile. Sophie is to be manipulated as mercilessly by her mother as is Emile by his tutor. Both "educators" are to seek to imprint habits on the developing bodies and minds of their charges, for Sophie and Emile are only able, by virtue of their "identical" formlessness, to absorb lessons experientially. They are incapable of "learning" through an act of reason or will.

---

[23]   The best-known episode illustrating the need to use experience rather than reasoning to teach a child involves the tutor's secretly destroying Emile's bean plants to have his charge "experience" the foundational notion of property (330–33).

[24]   Liselotte Steinbrügge, *The Moral Sex: Woman's Nature in the French Enlightenment* (New York: Oxford University Press, 1995), 56.

The ultimate goals of the two educations are of course complementary, that is to say, quite different. Young Emile is to be active and free roaming in order to exercise his curiosity for future use, once his reason has developed; Sophie is to learn stillness, patience, and obedience, qualities designed both to fit her culture's expectations and to counter certain specifically "female" qualities she is said to develop fully only at puberty (innate coquetry is prominent among these). But while Rousseau attacks educated or even excessively clever women at several points in this work (declaring of Ninon de Lenclos that he would have her neither as his friend—*mon ami*, in the male form—nor as his mistress), he presents Sophie as possessed of a curious and active young mind (736). He encourages his parent–readers to act as do Sophie's mother and father when their daughter asks them questions, for these ideal parents respond rather than ignoring their daughter or attempting to suppress her interest in "the little of the world that she has seen" (749). The verb "to see" is to be taken quite literally, for Rousseau has already specified that Sophie's mind is in no way to be formed by reading about others' experiences. She is in other words to be given no access to books. Why indeed, Rousseau asks, are parents in such a hurry to teach girls to read and write, when their young charges will not soon be in need of this knowledge for running a household—the only correct use, we understand, to which a woman is to put such knowledge? (708).

This last assumption was far from universal among eighteenth-century writers on the subject of childhood education for girls, of course. Abbé Le Moré, author of the *Institutional Principles, or How to Raise Children* (1774), declares that young boys and girls should be educated identically, in accordance with their physiological identity: "I do not distinguish the education of girls from that of boys. I think that in both the moral and the physical realms, there should be no difference, or at least very little."[25] Le Moré cites a wide range of authorities—Locke, Buffon, Tissot, Fénelon, and Montaigne, among others—in support of the soundness of his nonseparatist theory of education. Le Moré was however no advocate for sexual equality; he was merely advising parents in accordance with the accepted belief that there were no significant sexed differences in children until they had gone through puberty. Le Moré does insist that parents take into account above all the temperaments of their children: "It is indispensable to study and to know the temperament of young people, in order to regulate their degree of physical activity. I say the temperament of young people because it is only at the age of fifteen that we are able to begin to distinguish the temperament that will dominate in a person" (55). The exact nature of the "very little" difference Le Moré would have in the education of young girls and boys is most telling in his advice to skip Latin and Greek for girls, as they will have no use for these languages. He does however

---

[25] Abbé Le Moré, *Principes d'institution ou de la manière d'élever les enfans des deux sexes, par rapport au corps, à l'esprit et au coeur* (Paris: la Veuve Desaint, 1774), 10. Future references in the text. Le Moré was also the author of a book aimed at helping young children learn history.

advise stressing logic for girls even more than for boys, although what might at first seem a protofeminist statement is immediately undercut by the explanation that these girls will need this additional study when they are adults. Women, we are told, possess "a more lively imagination than men, and the liveliness of one's imagination diminishes the quality of one's judgment" (339).

Londa Schiebinger's claim that Rousseau was engaged in "wishful thinking" in writing "Sophie" is thus something of an overstatement:

> Differences in mind and morals were connected to sex, Rousseau held, though "not by relations which we are in a position to perceive." Rousseau's argument was based on wishful thinking, and not on scientific evidence. Though the connection was at best tenuous, Rousseau insisted that the physical grounded the moral, and that woman's constitution determined her place in the physical and moral order.[26]

What sets Rousseau apart from his contemporaries with regard to "Sophie" is not his statement that innate sex differences are "imperceptible," nor, of course, his firm belief that men and women are destined for different roles in life by virtue of their physiology. He is unique rather in the details of his differential philosophy of education for girls—details that square with his tutor's basic philosophy in educating Emile.

This belief in the "identity" of children did not quickly fade away, at least not in works heavily influenced by vitalist philosophy. The influence of this definition of "child" is evident as late as 1802, in the work of the ideologue physician Pierre-Jean-Georges Cabanis, an admirer of the vitalists who admits minor sexed differences in children, although he adds that detecting them requires "an attentive observer."[27] Another late, and far more striking declaration as to the identity and the extreme malleability of young children occurs in a 1799 dissertation for the Montpellier Medical School on the subject of "puberty as the crisis point of childhood illnesses." The author of this work, Paul Ferrier, emphasizes that we all begin as a formless mass of mucous tissue:

> The primitive state of all organic beings is mucous; the animal is originally nothing more than gelatin bearing the stamp of vitality ... The individual must grow; and so it is the force of expansion that predominates in childhood, aided by the laxity of the solids; the action of the tonic force is perfectly subordinate to this expansion: it does not begin to dominate until the age of puberty, and ... it is principally this change that cures most of the illnesses of childhood.[28]

---

[26]   Londa Schiebinger, *The Mind Has No Sex?* 221.

[27]   P. J. G. [Pierre-Jean-Georges] Cabanis, *Rapports du physique et du moral de l'homme*, 2 vols (Paris: Crapart, Caille, and Ravier: An X [1802]), I:318.

[28]   P. M. [Paul] Ferrier, *De la Puberté considérée comme crise des maladies de l'enfance*, in *Collection des thèses soutenues à l'école de médecine de Montpellier, en l'an VII* (Montpellier: Tournel, 1799), 8.

The expression "gelatin bearing the stamp of vitality" (*de la gelatine frappée au coin de la vitalité*), although referring to the fetus, illustrates again the quasi-human state attributed to children in vitalist thought. We are to view these creatures as "potential" rational creatures; animate beings, of course, but in whom the human life force in all its specificity is barely activated. Full humanity, in addition to sex, will develop only by the infusion of vivifying liquids that occurs at puberty.

Ferrier's argument that puberty brings an end to childhood illnesses by its "toning" or rigidifying effect reflects a much earlier treatise by Joseph Raulin, *On the Conservation of Children, or how to fortify them, preserve them and cure their diseases from the instant of their birth until the age of puberty* (1749). An expert in the field of childbirth, Raulin earned his medical degree at Bordeaux before establishing himself in Paris, where he was appointed physician to the king. Raulin was a prolific treatise writer who published on such subjects as the properties of mineral waters, pulmonary phthisis (tuberculosis), provincial midwives, and the vaginal discharge known as "white flowers." In his treatise on preserving the lives of young children, he describes the inherent danger of a child's physiology in a manner quite terrifying to parental sensibilities: "Children's bodies are like sponges that everything penetrates, even the emanations of the noxious sweat of sick bodies." The usual, horrifying cautionary tale follows: "a child of six months of age caught the pox from a diseased female servant who gave him a kiss."[29] The only "cure" for this childhood state of "permeability," Raulin informs his readers, is for the genital fluids to course through the body and, in doing so, take the reins of the animal economy (and, apparently, provide immunity from the effects of the bodily fluids of others).

The age at which the first outward signs of this activity are said to manifest themselves varies according to the author, but in girls is generally given to be between 10 and 12, with full nubility achieved at 15 or 16. The precise cause of the "awakening" of the genital organs is much debated, but is generally given to be plethora, an explanation dating back to Aristotle. The plethoric model holds that puberty begins when the growth process reaches its predestined goal and the copious supply of liquids previously channeled toward the formation of bone, tissue, and humors becomes suddenly superfluous. Until this moment, the body has adjusted to the constant influx of fluids by expanding, with Galen comparing the growing body to the blowing up of a pig's bladder, with the significant difference that the child's skin increases in surface mass rather than thinning as it stretches, under the influence of the body's "nutritive faculty."[30] At puberty however, the child ceases to grow—its skin ceases to stretch—and its body therefore becomes dramatically engorged. When the genitals are finally full to the bursting point, they are said to expel their liquids—now highly sexed by virtue of the "awakening" caused by this intense pressure—back into the rest of the body, transforming the entire organism.

---

[29] Joseph Raulin, *De la Conservation des enfants* (Paris: Merlin, 1749), 7.

[30] Tanner, *A History*, 10–11.

This plethoric model of childhood growth was one point on which the mechanists and the vitalists agreed. The mechanists, however, had a structural explanation for why growth stopped at a certain point rather than continuing indefinitely. The Boerhaavian theory was that as the child aged, his or her blood vessels and bodily solids became less and less flexible. This "hardening" over time meant that less and less fluid could be impelled through them.[31] Buffon refers to the relative "hardness" of the structural components of boy and girl children's bodies as the reason why girls begin puberty first, in a passage that refers to the awakening of the "generative parts" by plethora:

> [Males] have more solid and massive bodies, harder bones, firmer muscles, more compact flesh, one must presume that the time necessary to the full growth of their bodies must be longer than that of females; and it is only after this growth is entirely complete, or at least in great part complete, that the superfluous organic nourishment begins to be sent to the generative parts of the two sexes from all the other parts of the body.[32]

While early vitalists such as Astruc accepted this view of the onset of puberty, the explanation that puberty was the result of a general bodily swelling that reached a structural crisis point was too mechanistic for later vitalists. Roussel is quite vehement in attributing the arrival of puberty to the awakening of mysterious "interior forces" that come into play at a predetermined moment in an individual's development. Plethora does play a role in the process of puberty for Roussel, who describes the prenubile girl's womb as small, hard, and flat, but while this organ is said to expand as it overflows with puberty-related fluids, Roussel refuses to grant that there is a corresponding filling of her body as a whole (135). He points out that women do not always look engorged just before their first or subsequent periodic discharges and that some girls start bleeding before their bodies have reached full growth. He argues as well that if our bodies were indeed regulated solely by such a mechanical, fluid-based system—if plethora were the necessary impetus to puberty—thin children would never reach this stage of development, and they of course routinely do (192–3).

The observation that puberty begins at the same age in most individuals in spite of the many internal and external differences at work on the individual human form demonstrates to Roussel that the process must be independent of the gross physical causes others ascribe to it. Like dentition, he argues, puberty is destined to take place in almost all individuals at approximately the same age, for if this were not the case, "there would be nothing but confusion in the organized world, and everything would be subordinated to chance" (224). Louis de Lignac agrees, adding to a later edition of his 1772 *Of Man and Woman* that although exterior marks of puberty differ and its timing is affected by climate, "there is nevertheless

---

[31]   The mechanistic view of growth was far more complex than this brief summary indicates; for Boerhaave on human growth, see Tanner, *A History*, 68–71.

[32]   Buffon, *Histoire naturelle*, II:490.

a moment marked by nature for each individual. One recognizes it by the force acting upon the delicate organs influenced by puberty, and by the affluence of the generative principles, that excite desire."[33]

Roussel gives credit for the discovery that glandular activity is the determiner of puberty to Théophile de Bordeu, who, in addition to his influential work on cellular tissue, was known for his *Anatomical Research on the Position and Action of the Glands* (1751). In this important work, Bordeu argues against the mechanistic theory that the glands are manipulated into secreting fluids by the action of bones and muscles, citing as proof the following well-known experiment. After placing wet sponges in a human skull in the position occupied by the salivary glands, Bordeu worked the jaw and noted that no water was expressed. He concluded that salivation was to be understood as an action innate to the salivary gland itself, just as Roussel would conclude that the uterus "awakened" itself, rather than being forced out of its latent state by plethoric excess.[34] We are to understand that in Roussel's vision, the genitals "express" their sexed fluids, produced by the filling of these organs when nature sends its mysterious signal. The result is an astonishing transformation as much in the moral as the physical realm.

"Smallpox of the Mind" and Mental Masturbation

The end point of puberty—the sign that the child has become a young adult—is universally identified in these treatises as the first expulsion of genital fluids from the body, rather than back into the body. This visible expulsion takes the form of the ejaculation of semen in boys and the release of menstrual blood in girls. The previous definition of puberty (dating back to Aristotle) also involved the production of "seed" but was above all concerned with the appearance of pubic hair, as indicated by the Latin etymology of "pubescent": to become downy or hairy, to ripen.[35] Outward signs of maturation such as pubic hair are of

---

[33] Louis de Lignac, *De l'Homme et de la femme considérés physiquement dans l'état de mariage*, new ed., 2 vols (Lille: Lehoucq, 1778), II:216. Future references in the text to the original edition (Lille: J. B. Henry, 1772). As Lignac's reference to climate indicates, this all pervasive theory continues to be a necessary reference, and indeed persists well into the nineteenth century; see M. A. Raciborski, who declares that geographical latitude and climate determine age of first menstruation (*De la puberté et de l'âge critique chez la femme* [Paris: Baillière, 1844], 4).

[34] For how this experiment affected the debate on iatromechanism, see Roselyne Rey, "La Théorie de la sécrétion chez Bordeu, modèle de la physiologie et de la pathologie vitalistes," *Dix-Huitième Siècle* 23 (1991): 45–58. One practical aspect of this view of puberty was that young girls were no longer supposed to be bled to evoke a sympathetic menstruation, either when the onset of first menses seemed to be delayed, or when a young woman's period was irregular.

[35] See Tanner, *A History*, 7. Tanner assumes that Buffon shares this definition, although there is no clear indication as to which sense of *pubère* Buffon is using (*History*, 84).

course of little interest to the vitalists, and indeed a girl's first menstrual period and the first (preferably involuntary) ejaculation by a young boy are important only as signs that an internal process has run its course. The vitalists are far more interested in delaying these "expulsions" of fluid, and concentrate on the months during which the humors produced by the genitals remain within the body and are reabsorbed via the bloodstream. It is during this period, following the awakening of the genitals but prior to the external expulsion of the genital fluids, that these humors are said to be carried to all the major organs and in the process to transform previously uniform children into young adults of two quite thoroughly distinct sexes.

The most important organ acted upon by these fluids is the brain, and another point of agreement among these theoreticians of puberty is that the first sure sign that puberty has begun appears in the moral realm. Parents are to note carefully the moment when their previously contented offspring, whether boys or girls, begin to be morose and inward looking. Rousseau, true to his status as a pre-Romantic writer, offers the most poetic description of this psychic upheaval: "As the roaring of the sea far precedes the coming tempest, this stormy revolution is announced by the murmur of awakening passion: a muted fermentation warns of the approach of danger ... To these moral signs is then joined a humor in transition, and visible changes in the face" (*Emile*, 489–90).

The general cultural acceptance of this adolescent mental instability, and of its connection to the awakening of obscure desires at puberty, is demonstrated by the decidedly nonmedical *Essay on the Character, Mores, and Mind of Women in Different Centuries* (1772) by the poet and critic Antoine-Léonard Thomas, renowned for his oratorical skills. The *Essay*, best known today for Diderot's reference to it in his own essay *On Women* (1772), was first given as a speech at the Académie Française. As Liselotte Steinbrügge notes, this "agreeable" piece constitutes something of a summary of the debates on the nature of woman during Thomas's day, and is thus "just the place to learn which aspects of the mid-century *querelle* had gained intellectual influence."[36] Several of the assumptions about young women that had cultural currency at this time are revealed by Thomas's reference to an episode from Plutarch's *Virtues of Women* concerning the "Milesian maids." These young women—young virgins, we are to understand by "maids"—are said to have been seized with a mania for suicide, and to have stopped killing themselves only when the Senate passed a decree declaring that the body of any person dead by her own hand would be carried naked through the market before burial.[37] Plutarch tells us that this wave of suicides was popularly attributed to "a distracting and infectious constitution" of the air, but Thomas declares that these young women were "no doubt of the age at which nature, giving birth to anxious and vague desires, strongly affects the imagination; and

---

[36]   Steinbrügge, *The Moral Sex*, 35.

[37]   Antoine-Léonard Thomas, *Essai sur le caractère, les moeurs, et l'esprit des femmes dans les différents siècles* (Paris: Champion, 1987), 6.

the soul, astonished by its new needs, feels melancholy replace the calm and playfulness of childhood."[38]

Roussel repeats a provocative medical metaphor for this period of morosity: "One of the symptoms that ordinarily characterize this disposition is a certain taste for solitude and privacy that inevitably comes to young people, and that M. de Segrais calls *smallpox of the mind*" (212).[39] "Mental smallpox" is a strikingly rich image, implying as it does the "eruption" of emotional symptoms understood as so many behavioral pustules that are the result of internal forces at work upon the brain. As I will discuss in relation to Rousseau's Julie in Chapter 3, and again with regard to the infamous Mme de Merteuil in Chapter 4, smallpox was a highly useful disease for forming physico–moral metaphors in the eighteenth century, given the complex etiology assigned to it. Known in French as *la petite vérole*—with *la grande* being syphilis—smallpox was believed to be either communicated by contact with a diseased victim or present in the body from birth, albeit in a latent form. In the latter case, smallpox was said to be "awakened" by such diverse factors as stress or atmospheric pressure. Roussel's comparison of puberty to smallpox is telling in that it communicates both the eruption of a previously dormant yet powerful force and the quasi-pathological nature of this awakening.

The dangers inherent in the process of puberty are painted with stark colors in these works, as befits the writers' propagandistic imperative. In his discussion of the possible illnesses accompanying female puberty, Daignan "limits" himself to "chlorosis, languor, nausea, loss of appetite, melancholy" (I:198).[40] For Daignan, it was the overall physical health of the young person entering puberty that determined the eventual outcome. He tells his readers that if a child is of an inactive, weak nature, the overabundant humidity that results from pubescent plethora will "soak" the solids, slowing down circulation. The plethoric fluid will then be converted into "excrement," rather than into the "spirits" said to animate the fire of youth through their forceful action upon the brain. Weak individuals are thus doomed to an eternal infancy, Daignan tells us (I:110). Lignac in turn cites Hippocrates on the importance of avoiding such degradation of the blood at all ages:

> Hippocrates demonstrated with just a few words … that the return of corrupted fluid into the mass of blood deranges the functions of the mind and consequently produces mania. Blood, according to this great man, contributes so much to wisdom, that if you disturb its movement, and communicate some irregularity to it, there will quickly be an alternation in one's prudence, in one's notions, and in the feelings of one's soul. (II:261)

---

[38]   Plutarch, *Moralia*, 15 vols (Cambridge, MA: Harvard University Press, 1949–1976), III:509; Thomas, *Essai*, 6.

[39]   Roussel is no doubt referring to Jean Regnault de Segrais, who was a translator of Virgil and a poet in his own right.

[40]   Daignan uses the term *les pâles couleurs* for chlorosis, also called green sickness in English, or the "virgin's disease."

The potential problems associated with the swollen, fluid-filled pubescent body are many. The liquids coursing through these young, still unsolidified systems may be too "liquid" in nature, for example, and thus flow too rapidly for the relatively weak solids to bear. The result will be torn vessels and internal hemorrhaging. Or the solids may be too dense and resist the healthy flow of the liquids, said to be then forced back into the least resistant of the viscera, where they accumulate and cause obstruction. Death is a possible outcome, we are told, in all of these varied, complex cases. In order to protect their adolescent children from these threats, parents are encouraged to control all aspects of their offsprings' environment. Clothing must not be too binding and exercise none too taxing. The right kind and the proper amount of nourishment is said to be all important during puberty, as it can be used to control the relative density of liquids and solids and thus regulate temperament formation (this emphasis on the combination of the qualities of solids and liquids comes from the writings of Stahl, according to Roussel, 55).

The diet of the budding adolescent is one of the instances in which the parent must bow to the exigencies of climate. In his 1762 *Dissertation on the Physical Education of Children, from Birth until the Age of Puberty*, the Genevan physician Jacques Ballexserd recommends cold boiled meat for French children, while the parents of children raised in hot climates are told to serve their offspring a vegetarian diet.[41] Ballexserd goes on to comment: "The Supreme Being, in his infinite wisdom, made the foods best suited to feeding a country's inhabitants grow there in abundance" (190). In hot countries, we are told, one finds many plants, while cold countries "are abundantly supplied with fish, other animals, and grains, that must be prepared with fire; therefore these cold countries bristle with forests" (191). Ballexserd notes as well that it is imperative to make children chew their food thoroughly, given the needs of "second digestion," or chyle formation, in the liver: "It is not always the quantity of food that makes for the most chyle, it is the quality and the degree of preparation that it undergoes in order to be well digested" (183).

It is however the child's "moral diet" that is to be tended to with the greatest care, and all the more so when one is the parent of a pubescent girl. While the first stirrings of sexual desire in all young persons are to be considered part of the natural process of puberty—indeed, as one of its first outward manifestations—these feelings are to be aroused solely by the sensations that accompany the engorgement of the genitals, not by external stimulation. J. M. Tanner points out an early reference to the acceleration of puberty in young girls by exposure to decadent activity (kissing) in a 1669 treatise by G. F. Rall (*De generatione animalium*).

---

[41]   Jacques Ballexserd, *Dissertation sur l'Education Physique des enfans, Depuis leur naissance jusqu'à l'âge de puberté* (Paris: Vallat-La-Chappelle, 1762), 183. Future references in the text. Although not a vitalist, Ballexserd emphasizes reliance on natural processes rather than mechanical interventions. In the *Confessions* Rousseau accuses him of plagiarizing "word for word" from *Emile*, also published in 1762 (*Confessions*, in *Oeuvres complètes*, II:575).

Tanner discusses Rall in the context of Martin Schurig's *Parthenologia historico-medica* (1729), in which Schurig adds to Rall's forbidden kisses such activities as lascivious conversation, and repeats the commonplace that (very young, we assume) prostitutes experience early menarche by virtue of their occupation.[42] By mid-century however these asides on the early stimulation of the process of puberty have become the centerpiece of treatises on the subject, with the authors adding far more items to this list of causes and insisting with increasing vehemence on the nefarious effects of such premature maturation.

It follows that these authors are also extreme in the moral "diet" they recommend. One important proscription is that against the consumption of novels, given that these works are said to inflame the young imagination. While the novel had hardly been embraced by moralists before the middle of the century, Alexandre Wenger notes that pre-1750 attacks on the genre were almost strictly ecclesiastical, while in the latter half of the eighteenth century the medical profession led the charge.[43] Wegner cites a particularly striking anecdote given in Bienville's 1771 treatise on nymphomania, in which the young "Julie," newly pubescent, is given inappropriate reading material by her maid, with the most disastrous consequences.[44] Bienville's treatise is, however, a manual for curing such problems, and he recounts as well one of his dramatic success stories, that of the "too unfortunate Eléonore," with her haggard eyes, yellow skin, black teeth, and twisted, deformed body. After visiting this poor wretch in her convent cell, he tells us, he takes her home for treatment and informs us that she is now not only married but also "the most beautiful and morally upright woman of her province" (123). In contrast to "Julie," the ultimately more fortunate Eléonore's problems are attributed not to novel reading but rather to an "elongated" clitoris and "uterine lesions"—problems more easily cured, we are perhaps to understand, than an inflamed imagination.

While the sex organs per se are not generally of great interest to the vitalist writers, Louis de Lignac does turn his attention, however briefly, to the role of the clitoris in women's sexual experience. He declares that the clitoris is identical to the penis except that it lacks a urethra, and that it is "the principal source of pleasure for women during orgasm." He also declares the clitoris absent or at least latent until puberty, at which point it "grows according to the more or less erotic nature of [a girl's] temperament" (II:196).[45] The absence of the clitoris

---

[42] Schurig wrote "an astonishing series of eight monographs, published between 1720 and 1744," including *Spermatologia* and *Embyologia* (Tanner, *A History*, 78).

[43] Not everyone argued that novels were anathema to young people, of course; see Martin Nøjgaard, "L'Education de la Marquise: Un Contre-exemple? A propos des *Liaisons dangereuses*," *Orbis Litterarum: International Review of Literary Studies* 57.6 (2002), 416–19.

[44] See Wenger, *La Fibre littéraire*, 11–17.

[45] The exact mechanics of female orgasm are not explored in these treatises. John Falvey notes that La Mettrie comes close to a detailed description of female sexual organs

before puberty would seem to indicate that nature was protecting girls from being accidentally stimulated, unless of course their parents are so lax as to allow them access to novels. Even Roussel, who argues that the timing of puberty is part of a well-balanced natural progression, insists that we should not underestimate "the power over our souls possessed by an infinity of moral causes, such as the reading of erotic books, fixing the imagination too long on voluptuous images, the burning memory of a happiness irretrievably lost, or of a pleasure only glimpsed and then gone" (213).

Le Moré as well devotes considerable space in his educational treatise to the birth of "passion" in one's young charges. His description of how the sensations our bodies experience of exterior "objects" give rise to passion is typical in its cause-and-effect: "Certain ideas, when presented to our mind or to our imagination, excite in our body, as a consequence of its union with our soul, a more or less dramatic revolution, according to our temperament, in which the heart plays a great role. This vibration of the whole body, and principally of the heart, resounds in the soul, affecting it variously, and in spite of itself: that is passion" (149). Such vibrative effects are particularly dangerous during the vulnerable pubescent period, of course, but are said to continue to pose a threat until the young person's temperament is permanently set—until, that is, the end of adolescence, at which point marriage puts an end to such dangerously undirected desires.

While the hazard posed to girls by such artifacts of civilized society as novels is the main obsession of these treatises, young boys are also said to be in grave danger, and for a longer period of time. Daignan explains, in an echo of Buffon to which an emphasis on the quality of the male humor is added:

> Nature needs more time and more effort than with females to achieve the full growth and perfection of the male organization; not only because all of the male parts are more compact, more solid, stronger, and more energetic than those of females; but also, because it requires more effort, more work, more action, and more elaboration to perfect the prolific liquor of the man, than for that of the woman. (I:69–70)

The transformative power of man's "prolific liquor" when reabsorbed into his body is exalted by the physiologists, as in Goulin's description: "The seminal fluid of man is the purest and the most balsamic [health-giving] part of the blood: it is, according to Hippocrates, a substance taken from every part of our body. During the delicate childhood years, nature, eager to perfect her work, uses this liquor to vivify and to fortify the being to which she has given birth" (133).

The most hyperbolic praise of semen comes from a latecomer, P. Dusoulier, who addresses this fluid in a rather striking apostrophe: "Precious liquor, divine essence, soul of the world, inexhaustible source of life, to which humankind owes

---

and their functions in *La Volupté* ("Women and Sexuality in the Thought of La Mettrie," *Woman and society in eighteenth-century France: essays in honour of John Stephenson Spink*, ed. John Stephenson Spink, Eva Jacobs, et al. [London: Athlone Press, 1979], 63–4).

its eternal existence!"[46] Unlike Goulin, however, Dusoulier is referring to both the male and the female "semen," as do Daignan and Bordeu.[47] Bordeu even argues that a female "eunuch" weakened by the removal of her ovaries and the resulting loss of semen is "not inconceivable."[48] Both are essential to health, and he goes on to establish that the loss of this humor through masturbation even has a more marked effect on young girls, and especially on their faces: "Its deleterious effects are more evident in their delicate traits, and leave at times quite profound marks; astonished onlookers perceive only a shadow of the freshness and color that belongs to young people in general and in particular to women."[49] The complex logic behind this assertion is important to note. Pubescent girls are said to lose far less *liqueur* when masturbating than do boys, but are more harmed by this loss due to their weaker constitutions. They possess weaker constitutions, however, because the female genital humor is less "vivifying," so they lose both less "semen" and a less powerful version of this *liqueur*. Pubescent boys and young men are said to be both stronger and smarter than girls due to the effects of the extraordinarily powerful male *liqueur* that develops in their genitals and then flows into their organs (including the brain). But despite the protection this strengthening gives them relative to girls, boys have far more to lose with each act of masturbation or premature sex in terms of development, for their *liqueur* is both lost in a far greater quantity and is significantly stronger than that of their female counterparts.

The greatest danger for boys comes from the long-term effect that masturbation is said to have on the quality of their semen. Goulin stresses that the young man loses not only the immediate recirculation of fresh semen throughout his system, but also the benefits of future healthy "batches" of semen, for masturbation prevents this *liqueur* from developing into its rich, thick, adult form:

> In young men, this liquor does not have the necessary consistency: it is a sap beginning to develop, but that will quickly go bad, if it is required to do more than it can. It is an oil that is used up imperceptibly; if one does not know how to economize it: in a word, it would have been an exquisite balm, but it has been deprived of its qualities. In one's prime, the seminal fluid should be thick, sticky, whitish, and possess a rather disagreeable odor. It becomes thick when heated; but it possesses this essential quality only if it is not altered, by a conduct capable of diminishing the integrity of all the workings of the animal economy: otherwise it is nothing more than a whitish water that is good for nothing. (133–4)

---

[46] P. Dusoulier, *Avis aux jeunes gens des deux sexes* (Angers: Mame, 1810), 11. Dusoulier acknowledges the extent of his predecessors' influence in the full title: *Advice to Young People of Both Sexes, in Which are Gathered the Most Curious and Interesting Observations of Monsieur Tissot's Onanism and Monsieur de Bienville's Treatise on Nymphomania.*

[47] Antoine, Théophile, and François de Bordeu, *Recherches sur les maladies chroniques* (Paris: Ruault, 1775), 433–4 (Antoine was Théophile's father).

[48] Bordeu, *Recherches sur les maladies chroniques*, 394.

[49] Dusoulier, *Avis*, 13.

Even a well-formed adult who did not weaken his animal economy by masturbating as an adolescent is said to risk a great deal by indulging in this pleasurable act, for his body is said to continue to produce fresh sperm and to benefit from its reabsorption, provided he gives it the time to do so. The anonymous author of the *Encyclopédie* article "Semen" (1765) insists on how very, very long this "humor" is to remain in the "testicles and the seminal vesicles." It is the thickest of all the bodily humors, we are told:

> There is thus no other humor the preparation of which takes so long, the flow of which is slowed by so many detours, or that is held in repose such a long time … All of the [other] liquors go straight to their excretory points once separated [from the blood]; but what a long detour is made by semen, what a long route it must take in the testicle and its network, in the epididymis, in the vas deferens, in the vesicles, etc.[50]

Providing of course that "we" do not, the author notes, "violate the laws of nature and exhaust ourselves."

Anne Vila notes that in *On the Health of Men of Letters* (1766) Tissot presents the scholar's overuse of his brain as having the same effect as masturbation: "The body, straining to keep up with the demand to send more vital resources to the favored organ, was forced to neglect other organs and attenuate the overall vigor of its animating nervous fluid, which Tissot considered almost identical to semen."[51] This fluid should be understood as indeed "almost identical" to semen, for it consists of semen only very slightly transformed, semen that has not had time to develop into a fluid of true use to the brain, for it has not undergone the rich process of transformation described above, by virtue of a "long, long" period of repose in the body. It has been prematurely "pulled" so to speak from its meanderings; the scholar might just as well have "spilled his seed upon the ground," making study an act of mental masturbation in the literal sense.

Lignac explains that this view of seminal fluid as central to physical health is by no means new but rather sanctioned by the ancients: "The importance of the seminal fluid for maintaining vigorous health indicates that it is always necessary for part of this precious liquor to be pumped back into the mass of the blood after it attains its perfection: nothing can replace it in us, for doctors in all centuries have unanimously believed that the loss of an ounce of this humor weakens more than the loss of forty ounces of blood" (II:113; Lignac may have taken this quote from Tissot, for it appears almost word for word in *Onanism*[52]). The hygiene treatises I am examining were obviously not the source of the link between semen and male superiority, yet I would argue that they do represent the acme of this discourse in their insistence

---

[50] "Semence, Economie animale," in *Encyclopédie*, XIV:939.

[51] Anne Vila, "Sex, Procreation, and the Scholarly Life from Tissot to Balzac," *Eighteenth-Century Studies* 35.2 (2002): 240.

[52] Samuel Auguste David Tissot, *L'Onanisme: Essai sur les maladies produites par la masturbation* (Paris: Garnier Frères, 1905), 2.

on the link between semen and male cerebral fluid. Pamela Cheek refers to the emergence in the early part of the century of a "language of nervous physiology in which semen and the essence of mental perceptual activity were understood to be the same fluid."[53] By mid-century, in the treatises on the hygiene of puberty, semen was granted the power to turn a formless, irrational, sexless child into a paragon of manhood—should his parents allow this powerful *liqueur* to work its magic.

Parents were instructed that averting the threat posed to their son by premature sexual activity meant limiting the development of passion in his active imagination. Le Moré recommends keepings one's male charge from all novels, poetry, and plays, not to mention alcohol and "too frequent encounters with young women, and with young libertine men" (157). He adds that if in spite of these precautions passion should manifest itself in one's male child, the parent should try frightening him into avoiding ejaculation by citing the loss to his health. The threat of disinheritance is yet another option. If these do not work, however, Le Moré counsels his reader to marry him off quickly, i.e., to give him a legitimate outlet for the satisfaction of his desires as soon as possible.

The eunuch is a stock character in these treatises, for the obvious reason that he serves as an extreme example of male-physiology-gone-wrong. Deprived of all semen, the adult eunuch is said to resemble boy children in that he possesses only the "seminal power" transmitted to him by his father. Unlike these boys, of course, he will never benefit from the "stimulus" effect of his own freshly formed sperm, and his body and mind are said to remain forever childish, soft, and unreasoning. He is not the least fortunate of male creatures in this regard, however, for the vitalist emphasis on humoral balance meant that the overproduction of sperm might represent an even worse fate for a young boy than its static absence. In his *Research on Chronic Illnesses* (1775), Bordeu describes visiting what he refers to as three young "satyrs." Aged 10 to 11 years, these boys are nevertheless clearly "postpubescent," for they are said to be constantly masturbating. The resulting early and excessive loss of sperm has caused their brains to suffer, we are told, for Bordeu paints them as stupid, sad, savage, and above all, capable of thinking only of physical pleasure. We are perhaps to understand the cause of their "illness" as congenital rather than brought on by lascivious influences, in that they are described as possessing overdeveloped genitalia, although this overdevelopment is perhaps to be understood as a result of excessive masturbation. Bordeu does not speculate, perhaps because he was not engaged in the type of propagandistic writing that the later vitalists would practice, and thus makes no effort to link the condition of the three young "satyrs" to a cause. He does insist on the strong connection between body and mind evident in this striking case however, by declaring that these young unfortunates had "melted, so to speak, into sperm; they took their individual character from the seminal organism."[54]

---

[53]   Pamela Cheek, *Sexual Antipodes: Enlightenment Globalization and the Placing of Sex* (Stanford: Stanford University Press, 2003), 110.

[54]   Bordeu, *Recherches sur les maladies chroniques*, 417.

In sharp contrast to the "pitiful" eunuch, healthy adult men are said to be fortified by a rich, thick stream of seminal fluid flowing to their brains (with some of this fluid also, of course, dedicated to the procreation of the species). The daily reinvigoration provided the adult male body by a normal amount of newly formed sperm is said to consolidate and nourish its solids, to irritate and stimulate its fibers, and to produce the characteristic "fetid" odor of vigorous males, as Bordeu refers to it.[55] Men smell, in other words, of semen, a somewhat "disagreeable" smell, according to Goulin, but said to be highly attractive to women. Roussel attributes the courage, or rather the impetuosity, of the normal young man to the buildup of rich blood that is said to occur when semen has been allowed to be slowly reabsorbed and put to use by the male mind: "He fears nothing, due to the boiling blood that pulses in his veins, and that, in attempting to burst the dikes that hold it, makes him think that he can do so much" (5).

But as is constantly stressed of the girl's first menstrual period as well, in order for courage and all the other qualities cited as masculine to develop in this young paragon, the first evacuation of male genital fluid must not take place prematurely. The subtle matter created in his genitals must be given no other exit route than by way of the veins, so that, as Dusoulier writes, "perfected, impregnated with spirits," they may "carry force and health to every part of the body."[56] The post-Revolutionary Dusoulier, in an exaggerated version of the mandate for the social management of hygiene that began to develop in the late 1770s, goes so far as to propose a tribunal "where each Doctor could go to declare publicly: *The sick person who just died shortened his life by excess of dissipation!*"[57] Gentler tactics include Lignac's apostrophe to his young male readers instructing them that sex with a woman will not feel as good should they choose to "anticipate" sexual intercourse through masturbation (II:239).

Recent studies of the rising condemnation of masturbation during the eighteenth century, and above all Thomas Laqueur's *Solitary Sex: A Cultural History of Masturbation*, stress the novelty of the degree of attention devoted to masturbation beginning around 1720 and culminating in 1760 in Tissot's *Onanism*. Laqueur refers to Charles Taylor's *Sources of the Self: The Making of Modern Identity* when explaining the sudden rage against masturbation at this time. Taylor argues that the seventeenth and early eighteenth centuries saw the development of a modern moral identity built on the ideals of self-governance and autonomy, in which self-control, rather than obedience to a transcendent authority, plays a fundamental role.[58] Laqueur accordingly labels masturbation "the sexuality of the modern self," the secret act par excellence in a world in which transparency was at a premium. He notes: "Seminal loss was not the new problem. It was a chestnut

[55]   Bordeu, *Recherches sur les maladies chroniques*, 412.

[56]   Dusoulier, *Avis aux jeunes gens*, II:215.

[57]   Dusoulier, *Avis aux jeunes gens*, II:112.

[58]   Charles Taylor, *Sources of the Self: The Making of Modern Identity* (Cambridge, MA: Harvard University Press, 1989).

of ancient medicine, and it could not have been what so disturbed people about the masturbation of young boys and girls and especially of women, who produced in their orgasmic exercises nothing but fantasy and desire."[59]

An understanding of puberty and its role in sexual differentiation for eighteenth-century physiologists adds to this overarching history of masturbation by taking the subject momentarily outside the realm of "self control." First, the loss of female "semen" was a concern, as in the quote from Dusoulier, who was to a great extent recycling passages from Tissot's *Onanism*. In the section of this work that Tissot devotes to masturbation in women, he does not specifically mention female semen but declares that all of the maladies he has attributed to men who pursue this vice are present in women as well, along with some specific to women.[60] In the introductory pages to *Onanism* he does not refer to this *liqueur* as specifically male, although the examples he gives of its influence are exclusively male. We are perhaps to assume that while Tissot is obviously most interested in the loss of this humor in men, the fact that he gives no specific "cause" for the production of the same effects in women means that we are simply assumed to "know" that seminal loss is always the root of the many, horrifying illnesses attributed to this vice in both sexes.

Rather than speaking to a generalized fear of masturbation per se, the proscriptions against masturbation by young girls and boys in the treatises I have been examining were directly based on the ramifications of semen loss. Rather than the only product of female masturbation, "fantasy and desire" are presented as the principal causes of the loss of male and female semen by adolescents. The question of what behavior is "natural" is also answered differently when adolescents are involved; as Laqueur writes of adult masturbation: "Eighteenth-century doctors also had almost no interest in the Christian taxonomy of sexual sin. They certainly understood masturbation as 'unnatural' but only in the sense that a physiological process had more dire effects if carried out under unnatural rather than natural circumstances."[61] But whereas an adult was considered to be "naturally" stimulated to sex in the presence of a member of the opposite sex, and unnaturally in his or her absence, the most dangerous agent of the "unnatural" stimulation of sexual desire in adolescents was another person. Parents are exhorted to keep their young sons away from loose women above all, especially in the insidious form of nurses or governesses, and a charming young man and his flattering statements pose a far greater threat to a young girl than the stray novel.

While Tissot devotes a section of his discussion of masturbation in women to the subject of the dangers posed both to boys and girls by unscrupulous *précepteurs*, his obsession with the loss of semen (be it male or female) is not shared by the true vitalists. They argue that it is premature sexual awareness that is to be avoided

---

[59] Thomas W. Laqueur, *Solitary Sex: A Cultural History of Masturbation* (New York: Zone Books, 2004), 21.

[60] Tissot, *Onanisme*, 46.

[61] Laqueur, *Solitary Sex*, 191.

at all costs, rather than masturbation, and that the true evil occasioned by this awareness is not semen loss but rather the interruption of a natural physiological process of maturation. Nature, it is argued, firmly intends her most vulnerable creations to remain ignorant of how to release their "seed" until she herself arouses them to seek out sexual activity with an appropriate member of the opposite sex. In a natural environment, the young person's "knowledge" of how to slate his or her desires would form naturally and only at the ideal moment, that is, when he or she had become a fully grown young adult. Civilization was increasingly making this ideal situation a rarity, and deforming its children in the process.

One important vitalist even argued that masturbation could on occasion be used as a salutary medical "procedure" should such disturbances occur. The reference is found in the *Encyclopédie* article "Manustupration" ("manual stupration," or masturbation, 1765), by Jean-Joseph Ménuret de Chambaud. Roselyne Rey declares Ménuret, who earned his medical degree at Montpellier in 1757 before moving to Paris, the quintessential vitalist. She points in particular to the propagandistic drive with which he contributed 100 or so articles to Diderot's enormous enterprise, including "Animal Economy," "Leper," "Lethargy," "Mania," "Marriage," "Music (Effects of)," "Transfusion," "Urine," and "Uterus."[62] The article "Manustupration" was no doubt considered an important contribution to the *Encyclopédie*, given the vehement condemnations of onanism that followed Tissot's famous work, but Ménuret was definitely going against accepted wisdom in writing: "*Manustupration* that is not at all frequent, that is not the fruit of an overheated and voluptuous imagination, and that is, finally, the result of need, causes not the slightest negative consequences, and is not at all an evil (medically speaking)."[63]

Rey notes that to the contrary "one never finds in Tissot an apology for pleasure, and even less the remark that in certain situations, masturbation may be salutary and legitimately prescribed by a doctor."[64] Ménuret makes the argument for the prescription of this unusual cure in another of his *Encyclopédie* articles, "Satyriasis" (1765). He describes this condition as a desire-driven state of constant erection caused by the over-production, over-retention, or both, of semen. Ménuret notes that the source of this problem may be a deformation of the genital organs (as with the young boys cited by Bordeu), but, he insists, we must add

---

[62]   Ménuret also championed inoculation, in his *Avis aux mères sur la petite vérole et la rougeole* (1769), a work Elizabeth A. Williams points to as one of the first vitalist efforts "to focus on particularities of age, sex, temperament, and the other 'influences' governing health and disease" in a manner consciously styled on Tissot's success in popularizing hygiene (*A Cultural History*, 223).

[63]   Jean-Joseph Ménuret de Chambaud, "Manustupration (Médecine/Pathologie)," *Encyclopédie*, X:52.

[64]   Roselyne Rey, *Naissance et développement du vitalisme en France de la deuxième moitié du XVIIIᵉ siècle à la fin du Premier Empire* (Oxford: Voltaire Foundation, 2000), 262, note 155. Ménuret de Chambaud's first name is variously given as Jean-Joseph, Jean-Jacques, and Joseph-Jacques.

as potential causes debauchery, masturbation, obscene reading material, libertine conversations, and the like, all said to lead in some cases to an almost habitual erection, for the over-irritation of the genitals leads to the attraction of humors that form a "type of semen" in great abundance. Marriage is the only "authorized" cure, but when this arrangement is not possible, Ménuret counsels a full slate of purgatives. As a good vitalist he is inherently opposed to such interventionist efforts, however; he adds that these so-called remedies can make matters worse. And to think, he reflects, seemingly in passing, that it is so easy to dissipate this problem through "illegitimate means."[65]

There is a fascinating if typically convoluted echo of this view of masturbation as a salutary activity in the first half of Rousseau's *Confessions* (1782). Laqueur identifies Rousseau as the key representative of the first of three historical stages of the history of masturbation, arguing that the *Confessions* most clearly represents the moment at which masturbation became the great psychic battlefield for the sexuality of the self.[66] A close examination of the totality of Rousseau's statements on masturbation in the *Confessions* tells a slightly different story, however. The first mention of masturbation in the autobiography comes, significantly, before Rousseau passes through puberty (i.e., before his first experience of ejaculation).[67] He tells the reader of his stay in a hospice in Turin, during which a young "Moor," said to be enamored of our author, attempts to engage him in an act of mutual masturbation. Having drawn away in "terror," Rousseau tells us, he is nevertheless witness to the results of the young man's exertions: "I saw something spurt toward the fireplace and fall on the floor, something sticky and white, that turned my stomach. I rushed out on to the balcony, more shaken, more troubled, more frightened even than I had ever been in my life, and on the point of becoming ill."[68]

This interesting coexistence of ignorance and revulsion is meant to indicate that, as a "child" in all the truth of nature, Rousseau's younger autobiographical self instinctively knows that such activities are forbidden, yet on the rational level, he has not the slightest clue as to the sexual nature of such acts. Somehow, despite his difficult apprenticeship in the city of Geneva and his subsequent, unchaperoned wanderings throughout Europe, this young man has managed to contradict the argument (made by Emile's tutor) that only careful segregation from modern society ensures the natural timing of puberty in a child. In any civil society composed of

---

65 "Satyriasis, Médecine," *Encyclopédie*, XIV:703–4.

66 The classic reference to the study of sexuality and the self in Rousseau is Jean Starobinski's *Jean-Jacques Rousseau: la transparence et l'obstacle* (Paris: Plon, 1957). Among the many recent studies of modern selfhood that include a section on Rousseau, see Jerrold Seigel, *The Idea of the Self: Thought and Experience in Western Europe since the Seventeenth Century* (Cambridge: Cambridge University Press, 2005).

67 See my article, "Innocence of Experience: Rousseau on Puberty in the State of Civilization," *Journal of the History of Ideas* 71.2 (April 2010): 241–61.

68 Jean-Jacques Rousseau, *Confessions*, 66–7. Kamilla Denman considers the role of homosexual desire in the *Confessions* in "Recovering *Fraternité* in the Works of Rousseau: Jean-Jacques' Lost Brother," *Eighteenth-Century Studies* 29.2 (Winter 1995–1997): 191–210.

educated citizens, the tutor tells us, a young man's senses are sure to be awakened by his imagination, and this reversal of the natural state of affairs means that his desires will demonstrate that "precocious activity that never fails to enervate and to weaken first individuals, then, with time, even the species" (*Emile*, 495).

That such extended innocence was at one time quite unextraordinary is made clear in an anecdote found later in *Emile* in which Italy once again figures as a place of decadence and sexual enlightenment. The tutor is explaining that if one follows his methods, one can easily prolong the completion of male puberty (again, equated with first ejaculation) to at least 20. He observes that nothing was more common in recent centuries: "Montaigne's father, a man no less honest and truthful than strong and well formed, swore that he was a virgin when he married at the age of thirty, after long service in the Italian wars" (*Emile*, 640). The most impressive aspect of this anecdote is that "virginity," in the case of Montaigne-père, may well imply more than mere inexperience with intercourse. In the *Confessions*, Rousseau declares that he had come back to Annecy from his trip to Italy "not entirely as I had gone there; but as perhaps no one of my age has ever returned. I had brought back not my virginity, but my *pucelage*." We are to understand that some point in the year following his experience in the Turin hospice he had lost his "virginity," or rather, as Rousseau carefully terms it, his temperament had declared itself with its first "eruption," an event that is categorized as "very involuntary."[69]

While Rousseau's presentation of his own sexual development in the *Confessions* possesses an idiosyncratic twist not found in *Emile*, he is nevertheless echoing a number of the physiological givens of the day even in arguing that he himself is sui generis. The proposition that there existed, albeit living in the countryside and thus protected from vice by hard work and isolation, a physico–moral ideal of young French manhood is omnipresent in the hygiene treatises. This young rural paragon would be fortified by, indeed literally filled with, his unspilled seed, but too tired and innocent to think of masturbation or illicit sexual activity. His female counterpart would be equally innocent and luminous. Having passed successfully through puberty, thanks to a dearth of licentious influences, she would be perfectly sanguine in temperament, physically flawless, and above all, absolutely ignorant of the mechanics of sexual activity—yet physically primed for intercourse. This liminal moment of perfection, of course, will not last long, as I explore in the following chapter.

---

69   Rousseau, *Confessions*, 108–9.

Chapter 2
Women as Bellwethers of
Cultural Degradation

The fortunate [Tahitians] take everything from nature … how they are rewarded for this frugality, this temperance! The blood that flows through their veins is *primitive* blood; the juices that separate out of it, and particularly those destined for pleasure and reproduction, make beauty bloom.
—Louis de Lignac, *On Man and Woman Considered Physically in the State of Marriage* (1772)

The "simple, wholesome" lives of French peasants—like the "natural" lives of Lignac's Tahitians—are celebrated in the hygiene treatises, but these modes of living ultimately function only as signposts, and certainly not as models. Far from encouraging their parents-readers to take up physical labor and withdraw to the country with their daughters, the authors make it clear that only a young woman who has been adequately sheltered from her culture's decadence while simultaneously enjoying the softening effects of the highly civilized lifestyle will become a true masterpiece of nature and culture combined. The delights of the prototypical young French urban virgin, she whose perfection is as much the result of her civilized environment as a triumph over its pitfalls, are painted in glowing detail by these writers. This carefully cultivated "rose" is said to possess far more sinuous lines than her "savage" or country cousins, far more expressive eyes, softer, smoother hair, a more lilting voice, and pale skin through which one easily perceives her delicate, pulsing veins.

In accordance with the well-worn metaphor, the glory of this freshly blossoming rose is ephemeral. Nature has not produced her for mere show, but to serve a procreative function, and parents are told that should this brief splendor not be put to use immediately, it will be quite tragically wasted. After a pause to delight in her beauty, the physiologists thus turn to the moment in this young woman's life toward which all this parental attention has been directed: her marriage, or rather, her first sexual encounter. The preeminent vitalist Ménuret de Chambaud defines this institution in all its physiological connotations in his *Encyclopédie* article "Marriage (Medicine, Diet)": "We understand marriage here to consist of the particular moment of its physical execution, its consummation, in which the two sexes come together in a mutual embrace to experience strong, authorized [*permis*] feelings of pleasure that are increased and terminated by the reciprocal ejaculation of semen, and cemented and made precious by the formation of a child."[1] By classifying "marriage" as one of the nonnaturals, Ménuret places this "coming together" under the aegis of hygiene. The "authority" that "permits" this exchange of male and female semen is to be understood as the medical knowledge subtending Ménuret's many prescriptions concerning this act—not, of course, the imprimatur of the Church.

Neither is "love" to enter into marriage-related decisions, for parents who allow their child's desires to guide the choice of his or her mate are presented as almost as irresponsible as those fathers and mothers who arrange marriages for reasons of money or lineage. Fortunately, parents who have adhered to the hygiene practices recommended in these treatises will have prevented the development of "imagination" and thus of "passion" in their young charges, and need not fear such messy emotional complications. They are free to specify where and when and with whom, and then to retire from guiding young persons who after this first sexual experience are said to become truly independent, rational adults.

In the first part of this chapter, I consider "marriage" as defined by Ménuret and developed in the hygiene treatises. I emphasize that while marriage is presented as eminently healthy and desirable for young women, it is also, from the physiological point of view, destructive. According to the logic of the two-sex model, the injection of male semen into the young ingénue's body necessarily destroys the integrity of her feminine humors. The term *déflorer* captures this process as the vitalists envision it in all its complexity. What is "taken" from the young girl is not only her stunning virginal beauty (her "flowering") but also her "freshness." She passes from spring to summer, with the latter understood as the productive adult years during which she is far less glorious but productively useful. The infusion of the "precious male liquor" so extolled by the vitalists is said to have some positive effects in that it strengthens her body and enlightens her mind, but this increased rationality is presented as quite unimpressive in relation to that of her male peers. Nor does her new rationality make up for the loss of her luminous beauty and youthful innocence, in the eyes of the treatise writers.

In the second part of this chapter, I turn from the cultivated ideal of French womanhood as personified in these treatises to the stars of the authors' cautionary tales: those young urban-dwellers whose parents have not adequately watched over them. Rather than blossoming into the incandescent creatures they were destined by nature to be, these girls are said to be physically withered and morally unsound, and as such embody the worst fears at the heart of the cultural debates on the degradation of the French nation. These poor creatures, however fictional many of their stories may appear, are the nearest equivalent to control subjects in

---

[1]   Jean-Joseph Ménuret de Chambaud, "Mariage (Médecine, Diétique)," *Encyclopédie, ou Dictionnaire raisonné des sciences, des arts et des métiers*, ed. Denis Diderot and Jean d'Alembert (Paris: Briasson, etc., 1751–1765), X:116. Elizabeth A. Williams refers to Ménuret as one of the Montpellier physicians who gave the *Encyclopédie* its "insistently vitalist cast" (*A Cultural History of Medical Vitalism in Enlightenment Montpellier* [Aldershot, UK and Burlington, VT: Ashgate, 2008], 121).

these treatises. The diseases to which they are said to be subject and the dangers they pose to their potential mates and offspring must, we are told, be avoided at all costs, for a cure is next to impossible and the fate of European civilization is at stake. There are thus three categories of young women who populate these treatises: innocent county girls; corrupt city girls; and protected city girls. Only this last group is presented as the "cure" for what ails French culture, for while country girls may be guaranteed a healthy life characterized by hard physical activity and the complete lack of access to influences such as novels, they will never exhibit the exhilarating charms attributed to their protected city peers. Not every writer on puberty was willing to paint such an Edenic vision of French peasant life, even in the interest of attacking the lifestyle of wealthy eighteenth-century urbanites, but these exceptions should not mask the important consensus in these works as to the most pathetic victim of the ills of civilization: the unprotected urban girl whose path to womanhood is twisted by the decadent forces at work upon her.

Defloration, Enlightenment, and Masculinization

However much vitalism may have contributed to the eighteenth-century cult of motherhood, adult women are of much less theoretical interest to the vitalists than are their younger, virginal counterparts. The long period of (relative) physiological and moral stability said to follow puberty and "marriage" is simply too static to interest theorists for whom variability is the key characteristic of living beings. Women as spouses and mothers, however active they may be in the hard work of perpetuating the species, exhibit much less of the glandular action (nursing aside) and none of the transformative excitement at the heart of the vitalist reformulation of medical theory. By engaging in the act of sexual procreation, the ingénue loses her metaphorical significance, for the dichotomy of nature and culture—those extremes at the very heart of the Enlightenment—are nowhere more dramatically represented than in the young virgin's brief balancing act as she moves from childhood to sexually active womanhood.

The following passage by a P. Virard (*Essay on the Health of Nubile Girls*, 1776) is worth quoting at length in this context, both for its sweeping view of the process by which a girl child becomes a young woman and for the emotional excesses he reaches in describing the desired results of this difficult transformation. Virard defines the "nubile girls" of his title as those who are "ready to marry, that is, to be inseminated [*fécondées*], to become mothers."[2] He gives as the first sign of developing nubility in girls the mental disturbance that, as always, is said to indicate the onset of puberty:

---

[2]   P. Virard, *Essai sur la santé des filles nubiles* (London: Monory, 1776), v. Future references in the text. The *Essay* was republished in 1779 and an Italian translation was printed in 1794.

[They become] pale, dreamy, melancholic, bored by everything, and principally by that which used to amuse them the most; they seek solitude, then comes loss of appetite, digestion becomes difficult; they even sometimes feel like vomiting and ingesting strange substances; they feel a dull heat inside of their bodies that is very uncomfortable, their head feels heavy, their ideas are confused, anything at all tires them out, anything is able to cause the worst maladies in them; when, after a mild heat, felt principally in the lower stomach, there comes a tingling in the genitals, soon followed by the appearance of menstrual blood, that immediately erases all the uncomfortable precursors that had announced it, and replaces them with the most brilliant state of health. In fact, young girls never possess such a glorious complexion, more brilliant eyes, are never gayer or more intelligent, or more disposed to love, in a word, never more lovable, then they become at this point; and a learned Doctor has appropriately called the appearance of menstruation the dawn of the beautiful sex. (10)

One of the most important aspects of this young girl's beauty is the fullness or "liquid" quality of her body as a whole. While Virard points to the dangers inherent in this volatile physical state, Guillaume Daignan emphasizes how this "fluidity" adds to the beauty of his physiological ideal. As she approaches puberty, "The fine, soft, well nourished, smooth skin of this young girl, watered by humors that are sweet and well elaborated, and by a rich, well distributed blood, results in the soft mixture of lily and roses that is the best complexion." We are told that with time, this young girl's "interior dispositions," functioning "in unison with her body's functions," will cause the sudden "eruption" of her chest, an outward confirmation that "nature's vow has been accomplished." In other words, the perfect ingénue has been born:

From this moment on, all the young girl's charms reach their highest degree of perfection. Her countenance is more noble, her bearing more assured, her mind is more open and reflective, her voice more melodious, her gaze more tender, her manner more attractive; at last, by the happy conjunction of all the qualities of body and mind that she has taken on, she possesses the playfulness, the grace, and the laughter that captivate hearts.[3]

Despite Daignan's reference to this young woman's increasingly "open and reflective" mind, the female brain's lack of development compared to that of young men is a universal in these treatises. An extreme example of woman's supposed mental inferiority is found in *Emile*, but Rousseau's stance is not as unusual in its details as the wide dissemination of this educational treatise has perhaps made it appear. In agreeing with the commonplace conclusion that women experience very little mental development following their "second birth" at puberty, Rousseau evokes the eunuchs so often used as counter examples of normal male development in that they are said to produce none of the fresh sperm destined by nature to

---

[3]   Guillaume Daignan, *Tableau des variétés de la vie humaine*, 2 vols (Paris: chez l'Auteur, 1786), I:91–4. Future references in the text.

harden the bodies and sharpen the minds of male adolescents: "Men in whom this sexual development is prevented from occurring keep this conformity [to children] their entire lives, they are always big children, and women, who never lose this conformity, seem in many ways never to be anything else."[4] That this vision of woman was not unique to Rousseau and did not fade with the Revolution is clear in Paul Ferrier's 1799 dissertation for the Montpellier School of Medicine, in which he repeats Rousseau's dictum in more scientific terms, and more definitively as well: "In the [female] sex, the laxity of the mucous tissue preserves the uniform contour of the members, the nutritive system stubbornly retains its empire, and in this way one can say that a woman is always a child."[5]

Pierre Roussel explains the precise relationship between the female genitals and the brain when he explores "that brilliant epoch of [a young woman's] triumph, by which I mean puberty" (*The Physical and Moral System of Woman*, 1775).[6] In accordance with Bordeu's theories, Roussel's description of the birth of the ingénue's beauty relies heavily on the active expulsion of glandular fluids during puberty from not only her genitals but also her brain, along with the assumption of a strong sympathetic link between these two "central" organs. When the genitals awaken at puberty, Roussel explains, the brain is immediately awakened as well. The two organs then extend their beneficial nutritive forces to the other organs under their respective control (those parts of the body nearest to them). Under their beneficent influence, the Bordelian "cellular mass" extends and modifies itself, according to the qualities of the two humors in question. The brain, Roussel writes, releases a "productive" humor that works to round the neck and fill out the face, moving next down past the shoulders to elongate and soften the arms and fingers. The "softening" liquor produced by the brain is thus one of the many sources of the ingénue's new attractiveness to men, and seems in Roussel's vision to be created independently of the genital fluids, although simultaneously. The genitals, that "other center," cause similar transformations in the girl's "inferior parts," and the body as a whole is soon transformed: "The active principle or interior force that controls this development imparts a rarefied quality to the movement of the humors that gives consistency, heat, and color to all the body's parts" (81–2).

In addition to this overall "extension," Roussel lists the timbre of the young girl's voice and the expressive quality of her eyes as signs of her nubility. Her eyes are said to become filled with life (enlightened) when her senses sharpen under the influence of the vital fluids coursing through her body. This young woman's heightened sensibility, in the physiological sense of receptiveness to sensory input,

---

[4]   Jean-Jacques Rousseau, *Emile*, in *Oeuvres complètes*, 4 vols (Paris: Gallimard, 1959–1969), IV:489. Future references in the text.

[5]   P. M. [Paul] Ferrier, *De la Puberté considérée comme crise des maladies de l'enfance*, in *Collection des thèses soutenues à l'école de médecine de Montpellier* (Montpellier: Tournel, an VII [1799]), 7.

[6]   Pierre Roussel, *Système physique et moral de la femme* (Paris: Vincent, 1775), 78. Future references in the text.

places her in a unique category, for in comparison both to her child and adult selves and to her male counterparts at all stages of their existence, she experiences colors as far brighter, sounds as far louder, and odors as so strong that they become at times unbearably powerful, however innocuous they might seem to those around her.

One important (and infantilizing) result of these stronger sensory impressions in women is that they are said to be "happier" than "we" men, according to Roussel, who attributes this contentment less to the circumstances of women's lives than to their inability to concentrate on any one thing for long, so bombarded are they with powerful sensory information (29). Abbe Le Moré similarly links this fragmented perception of reality to the operation of the female eye, said to perceive objects imperfectly in that it passes over them so quickly.[7] As to the color of these highly sensitive ocular instruments, they are to be black or blue, with the former considered more expressive and the latter finer and sweeter. While not a sense organ, women's hair, and in particular its color, receives a seemingly inordinate amount of attention in these treatises, unless one is aware of how closely hair color is linked to temperament. Blond is the preferred color, as it is directly attributed to the effects of the moderate menstrual flow in women possessing the prized sanguine temperament. As Daignan assures parents, if a young girl begins menstruating at age 15, "without the eruption of menstruation having been prematurely provoked by hot remedies, by touching, or by lascivious images," she will inevitably be sanguine, and thus will possess "the best, the most brilliant, and the most pleasing of all constitutions" (I:230). Roussel informs his readers that his appreciation of Stahl grew even greater when he began to apply his predecessor's general theory of temperament to women, and noticed that Stahlian theory was perfectly suited to the subdiscipline of female physiology: "That which [Stahl] called the sanguine temperament appeared to me to be the most fitting and the most common in this sex" (xxvii).

That the supposed superiority of blond hair and light skin easily dismisses vast swaths of the world's female population obviously reflects a racist discourse of European superiority, but the rationales given for these preferences, it is important to note, are fully in keeping with such vitalist concerns as the readability of the body's humors. If a woman's body is to serve as a transparent sign system, capable of communicating its moral status to physiologists and laymen alike, a woman with dark skin is less desirable in that she is more difficult to read, if not fully unreadable. Evidence of the involuntary physiological act of blushing is highly prized as a sign of modesty in these treatises, as it was in the general culture, and the most common example given of the inferiority of dark skin in women is that it makes such reddening imperceptible. Rouge plays the same role and is therefore a sign of decadence and deceit, as Tassie Gwilliam has written: "The artificial

---

[7]   Abbé Le Moré, *Principes d'institution ou de la manière d'élever les enfans des deux sexes, par rapport au corps, à l'esprit et au coeur* (Paris: la Veuve Desaint, 1774), note to 339. Future references in the text.

blush is ordinarily read as a threat to the system of signs; it undermines and makes unreadable supposedly 'natural' distinctions, particularly distinctions between modest and immodest women."[8]

Rousseau, unsurprisingly, places a high value on the naturally occurring blush of the ideal mate he creates for his Emile. In the process, he presents mothers and fathers with a lesson in how to keep their daughters from any awareness of sexual desire. Sophie's mother begins quite early, we are told, to repress her daughter's natural gaiety, working gradually, carefully, and secretly to do so. From an (eminently sanguine) young child described as pleasingly *folâtre* (playfully exuberant), Sophie is slowly molded into a young prepubescent girl who is "modest and reserved even before it is time to be so" (750). The reference to the time at which she *must* be modest is a (quite subtle) allusion to the sexual desire that will well up in Sophie at puberty, at which time uncontrolled "gaiety" might easily lead her into the arms of a charming stranger. In drawing out this process of repression over the years before puberty begins, her mother is said to act out of "the fear that a too sudden change might instruct the girl of the moment that had made it necessary" (750).

The goal is not merely to create a modest young woman, but also and perhaps above all to prevent Sophie from realizing that she is indeed feeling sexual desire. Everyone other than Sophie herself is to understand exactly what her blushes signify: that this young girl is almost fully nubile, almost ready for "marriage." As is typical of the treatises in question here, Rousseau pauses in developing this pedagogical imperative to contemplate the titillating picture of Sophie's blushing confusion. He tells us that occasionally this half child/half woman will catch herself at play, and immediately stop herself: "it is so amusing [*plaisant*] to see her giving way at times to the habit of her childish vivaciousness, only to suddenly catch herself, stop talking, lower her eyes and blush: the intermediary term between the two ages [child and adult woman] must consist of a bit of both" (750).

While the blush's prized cultural status is easy to understand, it is less immediately clear why the authors of these treatises also valorize the presence of a "bluish tint" in a young woman's skin, indicating the presence of veins close to the skin's surface. Daignan's ideal exhibits "a complexion of ruby and rose, skin both white and well veined, supple members, an elegant form, blond, chestnut or light-brown hair" (I:231). The insistence on "well-veined skin" is a common trope of eighteenth-century novels as well, as I explore in the following chapters, and not just in France. As Christine Roulston points out, Lovelace admires the visibility of Clarissa's "every meandering vein," a narrative detail that Roulston interprets as a sign of Lovelace's refusal of "a transcendent reading of

---

8   Tassie Gwilliam, "Cosmetic Poetics: Coloring Faces in the Eighteenth Century," *Body and Text in the Eighteenth Century*, ed. Veronica Kelly and Dorothea von Mücke (Stanford: Stanford University Press, 1994), 148.

[Clarissa's] interiority."[9] I would of course read this detail, additionally, as contributing to Lovelace's attraction to Clarissa in that this feature reveals how well Clarissa's body signifies her exquisite femininity, including her feminine virtue.

The medical explanation for the visible presence of veins in the most beautiful of European women is that such specimens of femininity are composed of extremely "loose" connective tissues that allow their veins to come closer to the skin's surface than do the tissues of men or of "harder" women. It follows that the more "feminine" the tissue, the more visible the veins, and thus the bluer the face. Roussel adds that the highly "fluid" female humors are able to penetrate even the smallest of conduits, of which there are also said to be far more in women, with the result that a woman's bodily tissue offers "an infinite number of open routes to carry [blood] off to all sides" (63). That Roussel is speaking not of a blue color, but only of the pink tint of a woman's cheeks, is perhaps a reflection of his preference for glandular explanations of bodily phenomena, rather than explanations relying primarily on the pressure of fluids; it follows that Roussel's preferred complexion in women is alabaster tinted with rose.

A far more dramatic statement concerning the color palette of the ideal young woman's face comes from Louis-Jacques Moreau de la Sarthe, a late example of the type of author of interest to me but one who demonstrates a vehemence similar to Roussel's in stressing how fundamentally different women are from men: "Woman is not woman only because of a collection of organs and the enchanting attributes that we call her charms; for the naturalist and the doctor, her nature, her characteristics, manifest themselves in her morality as much as in her physical system … her constitution and that of man present at every point a series of oppositions and contrasts."[10] In the *Natural History of Woman* (1803), Moreau de la Sarthe makes the remarkable observation that the lighter, brighter, vermillion blood of young women is able to turn purple, yellow, and all shades of blue, at "the slightest feelings of surprise, of fear, of modesty, of love, or of pleasure" (I:277). In a rather bizarre form of racist discourse, he argues that the whiter and thinner a woman's skin the better, for the "more radiant reticular [net-like] tissue" possessed by such individuals is "more transparent and hides veins less well, the color of which, faded by the epidermis, gives off those bluish nuances that the charmed eye follows with such pleasure on the surface of the breasts and on all parts of the skin where the dermis is less thick" (I:168).[11]

---

[9]   Christine Roulston, *Virtue, Gender, and the Authentic Self in Eighteenth-Century Fiction* (Gainesville: University Press of Florida, 1998), 54. For a discussion of the blush in eighteenth-century novels, see Ruth Yeazell, *Fictions of Modesty: Women and Courtship in the English Novel* (Chicago: University of Chicago Press, 1991).

[10]   Louis-Jacques Moreau de la Sarthe, *Histoire naturelle de la femme*, 3 vols (Paris: Duprat, Letellier, 1803), I:14–15. Future references in the text. Moreau de la Sarthe (1771 to 1826) taught hygiene in Paris and was a passionate student of medical history, aided by his work as chief librarian of the Paris medical faculty. He counts as one of the chief representatives of the Revolutionary impulse to legislate public health (Cabanis was his mentor).

[11]   Sean M. Quinlan notes that the *Natural History* is significant for its "novel sections on female racial characteristics" (*The Great Nation in Decline: Sex, Modernity*

The "bluish tint" given off by visible surface veins thus joins the other qualities accorded to the young, postpubescent woman as part of the aforementioned general *éclat* that makes even the plainest of girls, we are told, suddenly of interest to men. All of these features are nature's way of granting this young virgin her extraordinary powers of attraction, and incidentally, of indicating to her parents that she may well be ready to begin her years of sexual activity and childbearing. The principal responsibility allotted to fathers and mothers at this point—their last charge as parents—is to choose their daughter's marriage partner and time her first sexual experience in accordance with the rules of hygiene. Parents are told that they have about two years to find the ideal mate after their daughter begins to menstruate. They are not to hurry the process, for they are also told that while the establishment of regular menstrual periods is usually the sign that a young woman may marry and have children, there is a chance that she may not yet be fully ready to withstand the pressures of pregnancy and childbirth. Her womb, that is, may not yet be fully developed, a process said to occur through the action of repeated menstrual cycles.

In his *Institutional Principles, or How to Raise Children* (1774), Le Moré is quite prescriptive as to the age at which young people should marry: 18 for young women, 20 for men. He repeats the commonplace that the harder male body takes longer to reach stability, and that "marriage weakens temperament, if it has not yet taken on all the necessary force" (67). Jean Goulin also gives the appropriate age for a young woman to marry as 18, provided that menstruation is well established and that the breasts are adequately formed (*The Woman's Doctor*, 1771).[12] As for the choice of a suitable partner, Goulin advises taking into account "height, facial features, age, temperament, and mores," although he specifies that precise equality is never the goal (157; Voltaire and Mme du Châtelet are cited more than once as a famously unsuitable couple, whose quarrels and sterility are said to be proof of the general maxim against the union of identical temperaments). Advanced medical training would indeed seem to be necessary in order to grasp the more nuanced points of physiologically based matchmaking, for as Louis de Lignac points out, the inexperienced onlooker might believe bilious and melancholic men to be suited for a life of solitude, but both types are, to the contrary, irresistibly drawn to women. As a trained physiologist, Lignac knows that a hermit's life would be for either temperamental type "the sad source of many illnesses."[13]

Waiting for one's child to settle into a fixed temperament is all the more important should he or she be interested in pursuing the religious life, according to Lignac. He would have all houses of religion imitate the practice of one mother superior of whom he has heard, who consults with a doctor to ensure that the constitution of the

---

and Health Crises in Revolutionary France c. 1750–1850 [Aldershot, UK and Burlington, VT: Ashgate, 2007], 132).

[12] Jean Goulin, *Le Médecin des dames, ou l'Art de les conserver en santé* (Paris: Vincent, 1771), 159. Future references in the text.

[13] Louis de Lignac, *De l'Homme et de la femme considérés physiquement dans l'état de mariage*, 2 vols (Lille: J. B. Henry, 1772), I:46. Future references in the text.

young women wishing to enter her establishment is suitable to the life of a nun (I:51). Anticonventual diatribes appear in all of these works, without exception, on similar grounds (see for example Moreau de la Sarthe, I:198–200; Virard, 35–6; Daignan, 167). Rousseau is among the most emphatically anticonventual, writing in *Emile* that "Convents are true schools of coquetry ... upon leaving them to enter into loud and lively company, young women feel immediately at home" (739).

Daignan does accept claustration for phlegmatics, those "cowardly" beings, as he calls them, "who grow slowly; with sad eyes, mournful and languishing; with fat on their bones, but soft, without firmness, and swollen" (250–51). Le Moré declares that parents must vanquish any child's repugnance for marriage unless they exhibit a clear vocation, or unless they possess "a complexion absolutely too delicate for marriage," with "complexion" a substitute for "temperament" and no doubt to be understood as equivalent to the signs Daignan points to as identifying a hopelessly phlegmatic type. Le Moré concludes by declaring celibacy to be nevertheless "against the order of nature," pointing out that most single persons "lead an unregulated, shameful life" (319).

Condemning a healthy young person to the sterile life of a convent should be understood as only slightly worse than marrying him or her to the wrong person for reasons of social and financial status. The very survival of the family line may be at stake, as Virard emphasizes, for although an arranged *mariage à la mode* might eventually produce offspring as the result of some "temperamental eruption," these children will of physiological necessity be feeble (40). The civilized state in itself is an obstacle to marriage according to Louis de Jaucourt, a doctor and the most prolific contributor to the *Encyclopédie*. Jaucourt argues in "Marriage (Natural Law)" that the natural attraction between the sexes is so strong that even "the beautiful sex," however shy, "invincibly gives itself over to the functions on which the propagation of the human species depends." In a state exhibiting "corrupted mores," however, marriage seems to offer "only suffering for those no longer capable of experiencing the pleasures of innocence," with the "suffering" in questions the risks and responsibilities of having children.[14] These risks are swept away in the passion felt by the citizens of "simpler" social formations, but prevail against nature in the more highly developed states. Jaucourt's main focus in making this argument is depopulation. He declares that France is showing the effects of social corruption just as did Rome during the decadence of this once great state. That Jaucourt was not a vitalist (he studied medicine in Leiden) is evident when he goes on to argue in favor of allowing young people relatively free rein in choosing their marriage partners. While he acknowledges that freedom of choice may bring on problems in some cases, he dismisses these exceptions in the light of the loss of "the few and all too limited years of women's fecundity."[15]

Six years after Jaucourt's article appeared, Diderot began writing his own, highly idiosyncratic reflection on civilized corruption and racial degradation:

---

[14]   Louis de Jaucourt, "Mariage (Droit naturel)," *Encyclopédie*, X:104.

[15]   Jaucourt, "Mariage (Droit naturel)," *Encyclopédie*, X:105.

the *Supplement to Bougainville's Voyage*.[16] The work is an imaginary addition to Louis-Antoine de Bougainville's *Voyage around the World* (also 1771), presented as material that this real-life explorer chose to exclude, for (of course fictitious) reasons that soon become clear. As in the epigraph to this chapter from Lignac's *On Man and Woman*, Diderot's Tahitians are presented as living in precise accord with the dictates of nature. The Tahitians, that is, obey the inner voice that instructs them on how to live, a voice that speaks in accents uncorrupted by civilized concerns. It is soon clear that nature, like Jaucourt, would have us produce as many offspring as possible. Unlike Jaucourt however, the Tahitians (or Diderot's Nature) do not allow their young adolescents to choose their mates; like the authors of the hygiene treatises, these islanders are deeply invested in having their children produce healthy offspring, and actively intervene to manage sexual unions and their outcomes. It follows that Tahitian society as a whole is constructed to maximize the opportunities for heterosexual intercourse, but only insofar as this activity furthers nature's primary goal of ensuring a continually healthy store of young Tahitians.

The *Supplement* has been read from a wide variety of critical perspectives, including Pamela Cheek's recent placing of this work in the context of sexual order and globalization (*Sexual Antipodes: Enlightenment Globalization and the Placing of Sex*, 2003).[17] As Cheek notes, the era of the initial British and French landfalls in the South Pacific stretched from 1767 to 1787, the period during which most of the treatises I have been exploring were published. Cheek delineates the five major themes marking the manner in which the South Pacific was incorporated into European thought at the time of these encounters: "the theme in climate theory that island nations tend toward liberty, the political economic theme that natural man has no notion of property, the classical theme of a mythic island reserved for sexual pleasure, the materialist theme that sex is an irreducible bodily need, and the natural historical theme of human degeneration."[18]

My own discussion of this work reflects two of Cheek's themes: the materialist theme that sex is an irreducible bodily need and the natural historical theme of human degeneration. The former, I would argue, has attracted an inordinate

---

[16] The original, 1771 version of the *Supplément au voyage de Bougainville* is lost; the work was first published in *Opuscules philosophiques et littéraires: la plupart posthumes ou inédites* (Paris: Chevet, 1796), a collection that included posthumous and/or unpublished works by a number of other authors such as Necker and Galiani.

[17] While many recent studies of the *Supplément* are, like Cheek's, written from the point of view of postcolonial studies, examples of the wide variety of critical responses to the *Supplément* include, on political theory, Sharon A. Stanley, "Unraveling Natural Utopia: Diderot's *Supplement to the Voyage of Bougainville*"; on philosophy, Guillaume Ansart, "Aspects of Rationality in Diderot's *Supplément au voyage de Bougainville*"; and on sexual politics, Dena Goodman, "The Structure of Political Argument in Diderot's *Supplément au voyage de Bougainville*."

[18] Pamela Cheek, *Sexual Antipodes: Enlightenment Globalization and the Placing of Sex* (Stanford: Stanford University Press, 2003), 139.

amount of attention with regard to Diderot's *Supplement*, to the detriment of our understanding of the latter and of the work as a whole. The centrality in this work of questions concerning the hygiene of puberty and the young girl's first sexual encounter must be read in the context of the vitalist hygiene treatises to be understood fully, and particularly in the context of their dire predictions for the future of the French "race." Diderot's close relationship with vitalism has been studied at length, and is most famously illustrated by his having made Théophile de Bordeu the mouthpiece for his dangerously materialist dialogue *D'Alembert's Dream*.[19] It is nevertheless important to note that Diderot reserved his serious proselytizing fervor for the enormous *Encyclopédie*. The wild, often comical musings contained in works like the *Dream* and the *Supplement* were never meant for a general audience, for they would certainly have brought down the wrath of the authorities upon their author.

As a result, Diderot's "desk drawer" writings exhibit little of the cultural anxiety found in the hygiene treatises and, of course, in the works of his sometime friend Rousseau. This playfulness is evident when Diderot turns in the *Supplement* to the question of how far Europeans have strayed from the "natural" sexual practices of the Tahitians. The topic arises in the part of the text said to recount a discussion between Orou, a Tahitian, and *l'Aumônier*, a hapless, albeit philosophically open minded French cleric. The Almoner gives a first-person account of his conversations with Orou, including the discussion that ensues after a night during which he has sex with Orou's youngest daughter—an act of hospitality pressed upon him by his host and committed, of course, in express opposition to the Almoner's vow of celibacy. These two representatives of disparate levels of civilization set themselves to discussing comparative cultural mores, and soon the topic of how Tahitian society deals with adolescents is raised and considered at length.

The Almoner asks Orou: "What precautions do you take to safeguard your adolescent [*adolescents*] boys and girls?"[20] Rather than expressing confusion at the notion of such limits on sexual activity—Orou's usual reaction to the Almoner's questions—the Tahitian grasps at once the European's purpose, and reveals that safeguarding adolescent children is such a vital concern for his society that it is "the principal object of our domestic education and the most important point of public mores" (983). During the two or three years following puberty, he explains, boys are required to wear a long tunic with a chain fastened about their loins, while girls must wear a white veil, so many indications to themselves and to others that they are to refrain from sex. One aspect in which Diderot's Tahitians and

---

[19]   Peter Hanns Reill observes that Diderot simplified the vitalists' ideas to fit his own philosophical interests: "[Diderot] collapsed all of their mediating assumptions into an identity founded upon the physical questions of how fibers were positioned and fermentation proceeded" (*Vitalizing Nature in the Enlightenment* [Berkeley: University of California Press, 2005], 185).

[20]   Denis Diderot, *Supplément au voyage de Bougainville*, in *Oeuvres* (Paris: Gallimard, 1951), 983. Future references in the text.

the vitalists are in perfect accord is the need to regulate as carefully as possible the pubescent boys and girls who represent their societies' future. While critical attention has been understandably focused on the striking differences between these representative cultures in the *Supplement*, the most important similarity I find in this text is that Diderot's "Tahitians" are just as energetic as their European (vitalist) counterparts in establishing strict regulations concerning the suppression of sexual activity among adolescents.

The outward, vestimentary signs that these young individuals are to refrain from sexual activity may be removed only when, in the case of boys, their elders are convinced that they are exhibiting "continuous symptoms of virility," and that these "seminal effusions" are both frequent and of a reassuringly high quality (984). The precise method for making the latter, qualitative determination is omitted, although Orou tells the Almoner that the appropriate age for a young man to begin the many sexual encounters that he, as a Tahitian, will enjoy during his life is 22, "two or three years beyond puberty," and thus slightly older than the European norm established by the physiologists (983). A Tahitian girl is to refrain from sex until she is officially declared "nubile," that is, until "she begins to look weak, to become bored, when she is mature enough to develop desires, to inspire desires, and to satisfy them in a useful manner" (984). No mention is made of menstruation in establishing female maturity, although "mental disturbances" and attractiveness to men, accompanied by the development of her own sexual desire and the ability to bear children (to satisfy men's desire in a "useful" manner) are identical to the signs used to establish a young woman's marriageability in the hygiene treatises.

As for the first of what will be for her as well many sexual partners, a young Tahitian woman is in theory free to choose, a practice that at first seems to pose a sharp contrast to the absolute authority given French parents. The parameters of this choice are carefully specified to the young Tahitian girls by their mothers, however, meaning that the parent effectively directs the union. The real difference between the vitalist prescriptions and the Tahitian process is that rather than making the choice of a proper "marriage" partner herself, the Tahitian mother teaches her young daughter the "signs" that indicate a healthy, appropriate mate. In the process, she hands down cultural information available to all (and inspired by nature) rather than contained in handbooks written by a few enlightened specialists.

Orou stresses that these maternal instructions are followed closely by Tahitian daughters when the latter participate in the fascinating ceremony that follows the removal of their veils. The uncovered girl is presented with an array of naked men who exhibit themselves to her "from all sides, and in every attitude," and her mother helps her to choose a partner based on signs not revealed to the readers of the *Supplement*. As we learn from a note supposedly scribbled by the Almoner in a marginal note to his manuscript, he considers these details not suitable for his "corrupt and superficial" European readers. The Almoner does express his regret at this suppression, for the inclusion of these signs would have allowed the French reader to see "to what extent a nation, occupied unceasingly with an important object, may succeed in its researches unaided by the resources of the physical sciences and anatomy" (984–5). While the winking undertone of this passage is clear, the social hygiene implications of the Tahitian practices are apparently to be taken seriously by the reader.

The most disturbing sentence attributed to Orou, from a postcolonialist perspective, is that in which he reveals to the Almoner the hidden agenda behind the Tahitians' eagerness to present their wives and daughters to the French. Far from a mere exercise in hospitality, Orou's insistence that the Almoner sleep with his daughters is an exercise in eugenics. The Almoner must swear to keep the information secret before Orou will reveal that the Tahitians have been carefully "harvesting" the French men's prolific *liqueur*: "While we are more robust and healthy than you, we perceived at first glance that you surpassed us in intelligence, and we immediately chose some of our most beautiful women and girls to gather the semen of a better race than our own" (990–91). The Tahitians also gave over to the French any young woman unable to reproduce with her own countrymen, in the hope that Bougainville's men might succeed where Tahitian men had failed. On a far more sinister note, Orou reveals that should the male offspring of the French visitors not prove to be "worth more" than their (pure blood) Tahitian comrades, they will be sent off as part of a tribute owed to a neighboring tribe.

While Cheek may be right in declaring that in the long term this response to the colonial enterprise indicates that "the Tahitians have already lost the contest," Orou's willingness to defer to the laws of breeding with no thought of racial pride makes the *Supplement* a representatively Diderotian exaggeration of the mindset found in the vitalist hygiene treatises.[21] Furthermore, his "Tahitians" are shown to have far surpassed the Europeans in their understanding of how to judge a sexual partner with an eye to furthering the health of one's society. That they are also willing to admit their own intellectual inferiority in engaging in the battle for racial optimization may not be such a limitation as it first appears to today's "enlightened" readers. However lubriciously tongue-in-cheek—not to mention racist—we may find Diderot's presentation of Tahitian culture, we are obviously also expected to laugh at those European parents not allowed to (or inclined to) make a minute inspection of the nude body and the semen of their daughter's potential mate, however crucial this choice is said to be to the future of one's family and indeed of one's culture.

But while Tahitian men may be examined in the manner of livestock before they are given the honor of deflowering a Tahitian virgin, it is important to note that Tahitian society as imagined by Diderot is at heart a patriarchy. Wilda Anderson has argued that hidden within the *Supplement*—in plain sight—is the reality that the dominant members of this fictionalized Tahitian society are those older men who have accumulated the most wives and children.[22] The "freedom"

---

21   Cheek, *Sexual Antipodes*, 182.

22   Wilda Anderson, *Diderot's Dream* (Baltimore: Johns Hopkins University Press, 1990), 127–67.

that the Tahitian men and women nevertheless possess, Anderson argues, is the result of their lack of enslavement to the civilized "passions" of the Europeans. It is this "disease"—"love" understood as an irrational motive in choosing a sexual partner—that is the most insidious of the disastrous effects the Europeans are said to have on the Tahitians, in a different section of the *Supplement* attributed to an observer quite unimpressed with his fellow Tahitians' willingness to engage in eugenic experiments.

The evidence that the Europeans are communicating this civilized "germ" to the Tahitians comes in the portion of the work given the title "The Old Man's Adieux." In this fictional monologue, a Tahitian elder complains bitterly that the women of his island have become "insane" in the arms of Bougainville's men. They have become, that is, "inflamed" with love and jealousy, emotions previously absent from Tahitian society.[23] The subtitle of the *Supplement*—"Dialogue between A. and B. on the Disadvantage of Attaching Moral Ideas to Certain Physical Actions Which Do Not Entail Them"—both sums up the old man's diatribe and echoes the principal concerns of the authors of treatises on adolescent hygiene. If the French are able to "communicate" this disease, it is because it is already hard at work decimating the morals of their own culture. Diderot's subtitle expresses both the goal of the vitalists and the principal problems they believed themselves to be facing: How does one present the eminently reasonable dictates of the hygiene of sexuality to readers imbued with the moral trappings of Catholicism and the snobbery of their social status, and inclined to accept love as a legitimate concern?

By appealing to their desire to perpetuate their family, in great part, and by avoiding explicitly anti-Catholic statements to the extent possible. "Shocking" suggestions that might seem better suited for the *Supplement* nevertheless make their way into the treatises; for example, although parents are not explicitly encouraged to sniff at their daughters' suitors, a young man's "atmosphere," or more properly, his odor, is said to serve as a sign of his virility. Moreau de la Sarthe, as is often the case, perhaps due to the late date of his work, develops this theme most fully. He informs his readers that the odor peculiar to any individual is a composite smell "comprised of one's volatilized debris, one's sweat, and one's emanations" (I:130). Moreau declares that an individual's odor carries, of course, "a sexual stamp," and that bathing in the "atmosphere" exuded by the opposite sex is imperative to maintaining the health of fully formed adults.

In the 1789 *Research on the Vapors*, Joseph Bressy, a Montpellier doctor, even advises men to share a bed with their wives or risk mental disturbances, for while men are said to smell of sperm, their wives' possess a "feminine" smell. This odor develops, of course, only at puberty, and is connected to the production of womb-related liquids, be these excreted through the vagina or absorbed into the body and

---

[23]   Cheek reads this passage as a reference to the Tahitian women's having adopted, or rather having been "infected by," certain "perverse" and/or "criminal" passions (*Sexual Antipodes*, 178); I read the passage as a reference to heightened passion leading to a desire for exclusivity, understood as contrary to the laws governing Tahitian sexual practice.

released through the pores. Like men, women are said to benefit from exposure to the atmosphere of the opposite sex, but also from the influence of the odor of other women, as when Bressy prescribes a possible cure for amenorrhea: "The young women and girls of the Southern Provinces are perhaps right to borrow the shirts worn by their menstruating friends, when they themselves are late; there is some sort of yeast left behind on the shirt, that insinuates itself into the pores."[24]

Despite this recommendation, and as ever in these treatises, the influence of female fluids pales in comparison to the power of male sperm to create an *aura seminalis*. As late as 1823, the ideologue physician Julien-Joseph Virey refers to the strong odor of healthy, intact men as a sign of intelligence, frankness, simplicity, and magnanimousness, all of which can be attributed to the sperm absorbed into their bodies (*On Woman Considered from a Physiological, Moral, and Literary Perspective*). Virey adds that the young girl takes on this manly characteristic when she becomes sexually active: "This odor is so much the effect of reabsorbed sperm that the young virgin, whose sweat is almost odorless, acquires a noticeable smell after she has submitted several times to the approaches of a man."[25] Virey agrees with the commonplace observations that the absorption of sperm makes married women more self-assured than virgins, and adds that the overexposure experienced by prostitutes causes them to become positively manly (*hommasses*). Virey even proposes that women who routinely work alongside men in less questionable professions develop "manly" attributes, one assumes through less invasive, airborne pathways.

Lignac declares that a change in a young woman's odor is the best possible clue to detecting loss of virginity outside of marriage. He admits that only the most sensitive nose would be able to distinguish this difference, citing as an example a blind man whose highly developed sense of smell allowed him to discern that his daughter was no longer a virgin (II:331–2). Lignac's reference to the extraordinary difficulty in establishing loss of virginity in a young girl reflects Enlightened French scientific opinion. In the 1765 *Encyclopédie* article "Virginity," Jaucourt cites Buffon as the definitive authority on the speciousness of such pseudo-proofs of virginity as the presence of a hymen (as does Lignac). Liselotte Steinbrügge's comment on the *Encyclopédie* articles devoted to women certainly applies here: "To a great extent, the *Encyclopédie* treats female physiology and maladies with strict medical matter-of-factness … This is true even in those cases which seem most open to all manner of misogynist speculation."[26]

While the writers of the hygiene treatises present themselves as working to dispel persistent cultural myths about human sexuality, their many references

---

[24]   Joseph Bressy, *Recherches sur les vapeurs* (London: 1789), 104. Future references in the text.

[25]   Julien-Joseph Virey, *De la femme sous ses rapports physiologique, moral, et littéraire*, 2nd ed. (Brussels: Wahlen, 1826), 187.

[26]   Liselotte Steinbrügge, *The Moral Sex: Woman's Nature in the French Enlightenment* (New York: Oxford University Press, 1995), 27.

to the increased mental alertness and acuity said to follow the awakening of sexual desire in young women is often accompanied by a reference to one of the most long-lasting and influential of such myths: the folk tradition that defloration awakens the minds of young girls [*fait venir l'esprit aux filles*]. Daignan explains this phenomenon, displacing it from sexual activity to the action of puberty on the mind, by observing that at the height of nubility a "multitude of nerves" radiate out of the uterus, and communicate with the abdominal nervous system (*le grand sympathique, trisplanchnique*), in so intense a manner that the uterus becomes "implicated in almost all of a woman's reactions and feelings" (I:270). He then makes a direct, corrective reference to the folk tradition in question, attributing to the action of this connection "that tender melancholy, those sudden talents that ferment and then suddenly break through in many girls around the time of puberty (and because of which they used to say that enlightenment came to them) [*d'où l'on a dit que l'esprit leur venait alors*]" (I:271).

The folk origins of this belief in the intellectual benefits of defloration are reflected in the literary use of this trope by Jean de La Fontaine. His "Comment l'esprit vient aux filles" (1674) is among the best-known literary examples of *déniaisement*, or the "removal of foolishness by sex" (La Fontaine's title is difficult to translate; one English edition gives it as "The Progress of Wit"). The "fille" in question is the virginal, idiotic Lise, who goes to the "school" of sexual activity:

> Before she went to this school,
> Lise was nothing but a miserable gosling.
> To sew and to spin were her only exercises;
> Not hers, but those of her fingers.

The reader is obviously not being asked to pity Lise, given the generic conventions of the piece (her lower-class origins are part of this generic discouragement of sympathy). It is indeed Lise's own mother who sends the young girl to "school," or rather, to the local priest, Father Bonaventure, whose very name reveals his clergyman's cliché willingness to "teach" such lessons:

> He wishes to give me such gifts,
> Me, only fourteen or fifteen years old?
> Am I worth it? the beauty said to herself,
> Her innocence increased her attractions:
> Love had no other maiden on his hook
> Who promised such good eating.[27]

That Lise gives her age as "fourteen or fifteen" means either that she is so limited that she does not even know her own age, or that, more likely, La Fontaine is referring to the age range commonly assigned to nubility in girls.

Eighteenth-century literary works contain numerous, often subtle references to this topos. In *Candide* (1759), to the hero's subsequent delight and downfall,

---

[27] Jean de La Fontaine, *Oeuvres complètes* (Paris: Gallimard, 1954), I:547–50.

Voltaire has the innocent Cunégonde become sexually excited when she inadvertently witnesses Pangloss teaching Paquette about "cause and effect" in the bushes—a literal *école buissonière*:

> As Mlle Cunégonde very much enjoyed studying the sciences, she observed, holding her breath, the reiterated experiments taking place before her; she saw the doctor's sufficient reason clearly; the effects and the causes; and returned home quite agitated, quite thoughtful, entirely filled with scholarly desire, thinking that she might be the sufficient reason of the young Candide, and that he could also be hers.[28]

Candide may remain rather slow witted through most of Voltaire's tale, but eighteenth-century male protagonists can also be the subject of enlightenment through sexual arousal, as Vera Lee notes: "The male protagonist of an eighteenth-century French novel usually begins his career as an innocent—but one whose innocence is based not on virtue but on ignorance." Lee emphasizes, as do I, that the relationship between sex and enlightenment in these works is nuanced, but still clearly present: "We find a constant link between the initial sexual adventure and worldly cleverness. And this link often implies a relationship of cause and effect."[29]

In a fleeting reference to this topos in Act I, Scene 1 of Beaumarchais's *The Marriage of Figaro* (1778), the title character asks his intended for "a little kiss" to "open his mind," so that he might devise the perfect scheme to catch the nefarious Count Almaviva, intent on "enlightening" Suzanne before her marriage. The link made here, a much generalized attribution of increased mental ability to sexual desire, is present in *Manon Lescaut* (1731) as well. Had Des Grieux not glimpsed Manon, he tells his listener—the famous "man of quality, retired from the world," and thus experienced enough to seize such nuances—he would have carried back "all his innocence" to his father. "Hélas!" he continues, such was not the case; he caught sight of her, at which point he, a young man who had never even thought of the difference between the sexes, and whose behavior had been admired by all who knew him, began to think of nothing else:

> I found myself suddenly inflamed, to the point of ecstasy ... While she was even younger than I, she received my advances with no embarrassment. I asked her what had brought her to Amiens and whether or not she knew anyone there. She responded frankly that her parents had sent her there to become a nun. Love had made me already so enlightened [*éclairé*], during the brief moment since it had entered my heart that I looked upon this plan as a fatal blow to my desires.[30]

---

[28]   Voltaire, *Candide*, in *Romans et contes* (Paris: Gallimard, 1979), 146–7.

[29]   Vera Lee, "Innocence and Initiation in the Eighteenth-Century French Novel," *Studies on Voltaire and the Eighteenth Century* 153 (1976): 1307–12.

[30]   Antoine François Prévost, *Histoire du chevalier Des Grieux et de Manon Lescaut* (Paris: Garnier, 1952), 50.

Given that Des Grieux is 17, we are to understand that Manon is perhaps 15 or 16; yet there is no timid blushing on the part of this young girl. She is well aware of desire and its power, an early awakening, in her case. Thanks to Des Grieux's sexually enhanced mental agility, and her own shamelessness, Manon will of course avoid a life of claustration, if not her ultimate fate of death in the "deserts" of Louisiana.

While most vitalist theorists viewed the infusion of male semen as a lessening of a young woman's astonishing feminine integrity, Ménuret to the contrary presents the effects of "marriage" as spectacularly beautifying for any young woman, in addition to its overall health benefits. This act, we are told, might transform even a sick young girl into a beauty. "The languishing chloretic girls, the sick, the pale, the disfigured," all are said to acquire immediate health, plumpness, and a flowering, animated face by virtue of intercourse. Even those who are "naturally ugly," we are told, might become "extremely pretty."[31] Given that the obvious rhetorical push behind Ménuret's article is to encourage marriage, understood as a well-regulated, monogamous sex life, this insistence on the beautification of young girls is understandable. Ménuret ends his article with the astonishing claim that nothing increases the health of a woman as much as pregnancy; indeed, we are told, there are women who are nearly always sick, except when they are pregnant and enjoying a degree of health "that nothing can alter, neither the suspension of menstruation, nor the uncomfortable weight of the child."[32]

Ménuret's graphic description of the evils awaiting young girls deprived of sexual activity places him back firmly in the mainstream of vitalist theory, although once again, the solution he proposes in the most extreme cases puts his practical applications beyond the pale. Referring to girls who are "spurred on" by particularly strong and precocious prickings of desire, he declares them to be made uncomfortable by the growing amount of (female) semen retained in their bodies. This plethora is not the only source of discomfort in such girls however, for "in addition, their wombs instinctively desire male semen; and when these two needs are not met, they fall into that chloretic delirium that is as destructive of health as it is of beauty, qualities that women [*le sexe*] regard as the most precious." Ménuret's claim that the uterus "aches" so to speak for male semen is unique but expresses a common belief in the "necessity" of heterosexual activity. The absence of male semen brings on "uterine furors," said by Ménuret to cause women to lose all sense of modesty and to seek by any means to satisfy their desires: "they do not even blush at attacking men, nor at attracting them by the most indecent postures and lascivious invitations." He suggest as a cure for those "thousands of cases when coitus authorized by marriage is not possible" the method of one "Rolfink," said to have procured the "excretion of semen" from a dangerously ill girl by some unnamed "artificial means," thereby curing

---

[31]   Ménuret de Chambaud, "Mariage (Médicine, Diétique)," *Encyclopéide*, X:118.

[32]   Ménuret de Chambaud, "Mariage," X:118.

her "entirely." Ménuret concludes: "It seems rather natural in certain extreme cases for health concerns to override all other considerations" (X:116).

"White Flowers" and the Etiolation of the Species

While young men are also susceptible to physiological and mental degradation, Ménuret's example illustrates once again that it is the ingénue who is the most seriously at risk. There is a contradiction inherent in this vision of women as the more vulnerable of the sexes, however, for one of the more fascinating consequences of the vitalist reformulation of puberty and sexual differentiation is that the female body serves, in many ways, as the model for the species as a whole. Women are by definition the more temperamentally healthy of the two sexes, for the male body is cast as a deviation from the sanguine ideal. The reabsorption of semen that begins at puberty may ensure the "virile" hardening of the male body and the "perfection" of the male mind, but this intense process of solidification is also said to obstruct the healthy discharge of other fluids in postpubescent young men. Even adult men, in whom this process continues to a lesser degree in that they are steadily "refortified" with reabsorbed sperm, are said to share in this undesirable rigidity. One of the many drawbacks to this loss of childhood sanguinity is that male bodies, with their less flexible solids and less fluid humors, are unable to adjust to the shock of an illness. Men are said either to overcome a malady at once, or to succumb just as quickly.[33]

Men are, of course, ultimately elevated above women by these very "drawbacks," in that they are compensated for these dangerous physical characteristics with what Roussel calls "a far more precious gift, that of strength" (89). When you add to the list of the influences resisted by the "hard" male body the effects wrought by an increasingly civilized (inactive, soft, highly sociable) lifestyle, the inability of the male body to adjust quickly becomes a relatively positive physiological quality. Men are certainly not presented as immune to such "softening," for the lament that French men have become increasingly effeminate over the centuries is common in both the physiological and the literary works I am considering. Bressy devotes his *Research on the Vapors* to the manifestations of this illness in men, although he does mention women at the end of his work, noting that the female sex suffers even more from civilization-related maladies than do his male subjects. Women, said to be possessed of "extra" organs—those of generation and lactation—necessarily exhibit more symptoms (134–5).

Bressy's primary rhetorical goal is to call French men to task by comparing them to the standard cultural point of reference, those fierce Frankish ancestors who had routed the occupying Romans, or their predecessors, the Gauls. He orders the once bellicose French men to "remember the character that made you in both form and soul superior to the masters of the world; soon the word 'vapors' will be

---

[33]   Moreau de la Sarthe, *Histoire naturelle de la femme*, I:179; Roussel, *Système physique et moral de la femme*, 58.

as foreign to you as it was to them. Softness, luxuries, enervation, pusillanimity, have made a sad Sardanapalus of your brain, become a weak organ that, used up in pleasures since youth, can now feel only pain" (84–5). Bressy declares himself nevertheless proud of his century for having banished ignorance and barbarity from within its boundaries: "I have offered the example of our fathers not to prove that they were more worthy than you are, but to encourage you to imitate them, insofar as their conduct was superior to our own" (87). Physical exercise joined with the benefits of a high level of civilization is the prescription for a happy life given in this treatise by a self-identified "Montpellier doctor."

The relative optimism of Bressy's 1789 call to action is typical of the Revolutionary period in its appeal to the possibility of renewal. Earlier vitalist treatments of cultural degradation are both less militaristic in tone and decidedly less optimistic. For the majority of the vitalists writing in the 1760s and 1770s, there is an unbreachable, if highly productive, dichotomy: "civilized" is the absolute opposite of natural, with the latter conceived of as fully healthy, but the former as a far sweeter mode of existence. The two can never truly coexist harmoniously, for whatever attenuating practices may be developed, one simply cannot have it both ways. One cannot be both a perfect physical and moral specimen and a highly sophisticated individual. The indulgent tone of the majority of these authors when discussing the ingénue, that sweet, attractive, and above all (necessarily) ignorant creature, conveys a cultural nostalgia for a simpler time in the life of the culture: the golden age of the Gauls, the Franks, or of Chivalry.

The most common (and obvious) point of contrast to the dangers of urban existence is the lifestyle of eighteenth-century country folk. As with many of the tenets of the hygiene treatises, this theory was neither new nor unique to the vitalist writers in France. In his *History of Human Growth* (1981), J. M. Tanner emphasizes the moralizing aspect of this theme in the writings of a seventeenth-century forerunner of social medicine, Hippolyt Guarinoni, a German doctor who studied medicine in Padua before becoming physician to the Royal Convent in Hall, near Innsbruck. Tanner writes of Guarinoni's lengthy study *The Abomination of Desolation of Humankind* (1610): "It is, if such a thing is possible, a book of devotional hygiene."[34] While Guarinoni campaigned for the benefits of clean air and pure water, he also argued that belief in God was more therapeutically powerful than the six nonnaturals: "Guarinoni loved the countryside and the peasants. He extolled the virtue of the simple life, and thought the *Bauerschaft* (farmers and peasants) both healthier and nearer to God (not that he distinguished those two things very clearly) than the nobles and merchants."[35] Guarinoni observes of peasants girls in the mountainous Tyrol region:

---

[34] J. M. Tanner, *A History of the Study of Human Growth* (Cambridge: Cambridge University Press, 1981), 29.

[35] Tanner, *History*, 28.

The peasant girls of this *Landschaft* in general menstruate much later than the daughters of the townsfolk or the aristocracy ... The townsfolk have usually borne several children before the peasant girls have yet menstruated. The cause seems to be that the inhabitants of the town consume more fat (moist) foods and drink and so their bodies become soft, weak, and fat and come early to menstruation, in the same way as a tree which one waters too early produces earlier but less well-formed fruit than another.[36]

In the eighteenth-century French treatises, rural adolescents are said to experience "natural" puberty, with Lignac most clearly differentiating this variety of puberty from "the type of puberty that you will permit me to call *false* [*factice*; emphasis is Lignac's]. This type owes its birth to dangerous liaisons, obscene reading, succulent foods, to everything that inflames the imagination; the other is the work of nature" (II:227). It is important to note that Lignac is not referring to puberty in the "state of nature," as will Laclos (see Chapter 5). The "state of nature," in the Rousseauian sense of the primordial stage of human development, is of little interest to the vitalists, who deal in practical matters of public hygiene. In referring to the benefits of "natural" puberty, Lignac simply means that when internal fluids act alone to awaken the genitals, there is little upset to the child's system. In the countryside, or in a parent-constructed urban cocoon, the young person remains relatively tranquil as he or she passes through this period of intense transformation. As Lignac portrays him, the young boy who lives in the country and thus goes through puberty unaffected by urban iniquity will develop into a rural Adonis: "Look at this adolescent, already vigorous, who exercises his body with labor in the fields; a light down is scarcely visible on his chin, his muscular arms gracefully perform the tasks he asks of them, nothing exterior accelerates in him the development of puberty" (II:228). He is, Lignac continues, like a tree in winter, apparently dead, but in which nature is working to produce the sap that will run through it with the first warmth of spring.

While this young man's city counterparts are deprived of his level of health and vigor, it is their urban female companions who are the true victims of the civilized lifestyle. That an abrupt increase in the number of "female diseases" should be understood as the clearest sign of the French nation's ongoing self-destruction is made clear in the preliminary discourse to Joseph Raulin's 1766 *Treatise on White Flowers*. Raulin's *fleurs blanches*, from the Latin "fluor albus," or "white flow," is now most commonly termed leucorrhaea, and consists of a whitish vaginal discharge (indicative of infection). The author of the previously cited *On the Conservation of Children* (1749), Raulin assures us in his *White Flowers* that the proliferation of this particularly insidious disease is nature's way of sending us the clearest possible signal that humankind is in a downward spiral: "It is principally this malady that is causing the human species to degenerate

---

[36]   As cited by Tanner, *History*, 29–30, from Hippolyt Guarinoni, *Die Grewel der Verwüstung menschlichen Geschlechts* (Ingolstatt: Angermayr, 1610).

and alarming nature."[37] Weak organs (the result of general inactivity), the mixing of the European "races" (*des différents peuples*), and the use of luxury products, especially those from the Indies, are all said by Raulin to have combined to make "white flowers" hereditary in French women, with heredity understood in this pre-Darwinian age as the effect of habit on bodies over the generations. As a result, a disease all but unknown in the fourteenth century, according to Raulin, is now seen in women of all ages, even the youngest, although the disease is—of course—especially virulent among rich city dwellers.

Although Raulin is the most rhetorically extravagant in his attacks on the nefarious results of the supposed epidemic of *les fleurs blanches*, other physiologists also view this disease as particularly symptomatic of a decadent lifestyle. Jean Goulin, in *The Women's Doctor* (1771), defines "white flowers" as a "serous humoral flow, lymphatic, viscous, white in its natural state, but sometimes green, yellowish, or blackish." This noxious, contagious discharge, Goulin explains, is often present just before or after a woman's period. While it is said to occur less frequently in young girls, such individuals may well experience this discharge if they are out of balance: "Those of the phlegmatic temperament are more often subject to this illness than those of a good [sanguine] temperament, who digest well" (111). While Raulin points to diet and lack of exercise as the source of this disease, Goulin ascribes it above all to an overly active sex life. He also posits a separate source for "white flowers" from that of the healthy flow of menstrual blood: "The *fleurs blanches* come from the lymphatic veins of the womb, while menstrual blood, properly called, is produced by the sanguinary vessels" (112).

In a different treatise, Goulin instructs his readers in how to differentiate this noxious humor from a light menstrual flow, or from the different type of discharge that results from overindulgence in beer by women, both declared innocuous, or noncontagious. The location of this last bit of information—*The Men's Doctor*, a companion book to *The Women's Doctor*—reflects Goulin's concern for the effects of this disease on husbands. He instructs men to be on the watch for these "pale colors," but adds that they should not assume the worst about their wives should they discover the presence of this illness in them (infidelity being the worst). The husband may well be himself the unwitting source of the illness: "One can be exposed to [this contagion] with the most honest woman, when one does not know moderation," or when one's wife insists on an overactive marital sex life.[38] Debauchery is found in the least likely of places, in other words: the marital bed. Like Raulin, Bressy, and Bienville, and in a manner as hortatory as the priests whose authority on the subject of marriage they would usurp, Goulin's work begins with a Ciceronian *O tempora, o mores*:

---

[37] Joseph Raulin, *Traité des fleurs blanches* (Paris: Herissant, 1766), vi.

[38] Jean Goulin, *Le Médecin des hommes, depuis la puberté jusqu'à l'extrême vieillesse* (Paris: Vincent, 1772), 241.

"Morals today are so corrupt, that it seems as if people blush less from being debauched than from appearing virtuous."[39]

Pierre Pomme, an expert on the "vapors" in women who treated an elite clientele, preceded Raulin in arguing against the faddish use of foodstuffs such as chocolate and coffee. Having earned a medical degree from Montpellier in the 1750s, Pomme proudly declares himself a "Montpellier doctor" on the title page of his *Treatise on the Vaporous Affections of Both Sexes* (1760), a work that includes an "Explanation of Some Medical Terms" destined for the nonspecialist reader. Although both chocolate and coffee are said to have their place in curing the occasional indisposition, Pomme, like Raulin, argues for their general unsuitability to the European digestive system, calling them "pernicious," and identifying them as nonimmediate causes (*causes éloignées*) of the vapors. These foreign substances act by "the evaporation of the fluid that lubricates [the nerves], that makes them supple and able to execute the vital functions in an orderly and untroubled manner. Will not blood and the other humors also be affected by such a constitution?"[40] The thicker secretions caused by the social abuse of what should be medicinal substances, we are to understand, leads to slowed circulation, a sluggishness that obstructs the viscera and obliterates the blood vessels. Ultimately the body becomes unable to absorb and process food, and the result is death.

The civilized state is as easily blamed for an unhealthy thinning of the humors as it for the thickening of the bodily fluids; either state is, for the vitalists, a primary cause of illness, in keeping with their resurrection of humoralism, for each condition is symptomatic of an overall imbalance. By far the most common evidence of an overabundance of bodily fluid in women, and one mentioned even more often than the dreaded "white flowers," is excessive menstruation. According to Astruc, one of the earliest and most influential vitalists, country women experience very little bleeding, and peasant women can indeed go two months with no period at all; meanwhile, "girls living in a state of softness and heat often lose blood two or even three times per month, which entirely destroys them."[41]

The quantity of blood lost by any woman during menstruation is generally said to correlate to the degree of civilization enjoyed by her culture, although different equations are given by different commentators. The production of a very small amount of blood, or even the apparent absence of blood, is said to be characteristic of both the "natural" lifestyle and the "overcivilized" lifestyle. Astruc goes so far as to question the "naturalness" of a noticeable blood flow during menstruation, declaring that rather than viewing nonmenstruating women as "sharing in some manner in the nature of men," we should see them as more eminently female than their bleeding sisters. He backs up this statement with a number of "observed"

---

[39]   Goulin, *Le Médecin des hommes*, 62.

[40]   Pierre Pomme, *Essai sur les Affections vaporeuses des deux sexes* (Paris: Desaint & Saillant, 1760), 30–31.

[41]   Jean Astruc, *Traité des Maladies des femmes*, 6 vols. (Paris: Cavelier, 1761–1765), I:12–13. Future references in the text.

facts, first from France: "We know that in general country women, who live frugally, bleed less than those women in cities who live in a state of abundance" (I:84). He then moves on to travel narratives, citing voyagers who have been to Brazil and Greenland as to how primitive women, like female animals, either do not menstruate at all or produce only a pale reddish discharge. Astruc concludes that the abundant bleeding one commonly observes in (European) women was not "instituted by nature." He concludes:

> This makes one think that there must have been originally the case for all women; and that those who have continued to live in the primal simplicity of nature have also continued to enjoy the advantages that nature accorded them; and that if the women from the nations we call *civilized*, are to the contrary afflicted with heavier and more painful menstrual periods, it is because the softness and the excesses of the lives they lead pervert their natural constitutions and multiply or worsen their infirmities. (I:85)

Roussel agrees, noting with the same assurance that animals do not menstruate, and concluding: "All of these facts strongly indicate that there must have been a time when women were not subject to this incommodious tribute; and that the menstrual flow, far from being a natural institution, is to the contrary a factitious need contracted in a social state" (197).[42] Offering a visceral explanation for the development of menstruation in women, Roussel blames the appearance of this phenomenon on overeating and the subsequent need to "rid oneself of dangerous superfluity by means of appropriate evacuations" (199). While men overeat as well of course, their superfluous humors must be expelled from different locations, for they lack woman's commodious channel. Older men are said to expel the excess via hemorrhoids, the young through nosebleeds.

That the human animal indulges in such unnaturally copious "feasts" is a result, Roussel argues, of our love for social gatherings. We stay at table far after our appetite has been satisfied; the natural switch that indicates fullness is, apparently, somehow turned off by the pleasures of sociability. Employing a comparison that makes the pathological nature of menstruation quite clear, Roussel writes: "In the present state of affairs, a woman is born with the disposition to menstruate at a certain age, just as she is born with the disposition to develop smallpox" (210). The belief that such anomalies may become hereditary as generation after generation of women indulge in unhealthy habits allows Roussel to explain away the existence of thin girls who, although quite abstemious at the table, nevertheless menstruate excessively. These girls' ancestors have influenced them such that, even in the absence of overabundant intake of food—the primary cause of excessive menstruation (*la cause primitive*)—these girls must still pay tribute to civilization's nefarious effects.

In addition to their reasonable diet, country people are said to be, as is evident in Goulin's young Adonis, much more active than their urban counterparts—

---

[42] Virey rejects this argument in *De la femme*, 11.

although here class differences tend to blur considerably, as the urban rich are compared to the rural peasants, rather than to wealthier inhabitants of the French countryside. Young country women are in general presented as working hard and as benefiting from this labor just as much as their male peers. Jean-Charles Desessartz, a doctor associated with the Medical School of Paris, attributes the extraordinary health of country girls primarily to the exercise they perform as part of their daily routine:

> What a difference between the force and health of village girls and our Demoiselles! Why do the former have such high color, such a rosy complexion, a constitution that stands up to the vicissitudes of the seasons … while the latter lead a miserable life … always dangerously sick when they are close to the state of puberty? In addition to the infinite disparity between the diets of the two, the village girls are constantly moving.[43]

Desessartz's *Treatise on the Physical Education of Young Children* (1760) strongly influenced the portrayal of puberty in *Emile*, and the dichotomy of country and city functions in this work in the same way as it does in Rousseau's far more famous pedagogical treatise, published two years later. But while the tutor carefully safeguards Emile from the dangers of urban licentiousness, the city eventually corrupts even his charge's carefully plotted existence. In the lesser known sequel, *Emile and Sophie, or The Solitary Ones* (1780), we learn that the couple has had and then lost a child, leaving Sophie emotionally devastated. They move to Paris in search of distraction, and in that urban den of iniquity, Sophie is unfaithful to her husband, who leaves her to travel in an attempt to forget his pain.

Some French physiologists were of course disinclined to accept that life in the poor, rural regions of their country constituted a bucolic idyll. Buffon was perhaps the most influential of such authors, for in his *Natural History* he declared that the malnourishment of country children resulted in a delay of two to three years in the onset of puberty.[44] In a footnote to *Emile*, Rousseau contests Buffon's claim by evoking his beloved Valais, high in the Swiss Alps. He tells his readers that while Buffon's "observation" is accurate, his explanation is not; in other words, Rousseau accepts the existence of this delay, but attributes it to the simplicity of mores in the high-mountain dwellers.[45] Pomme joins Buffon in pointing out that hardworking country girls do not always live in a paradise of natural abundance. Given their relatively fragile female constitutions, their nerves are often "broken," he says, or "weakened by various muscle contractions."[46]

---

[43]   Jean-Charles Desessartz, *Traité de l'éducation corporelle des enfants en bas âge ou Réflexions pratiques sur les moyens de procurer une meilleure constitution aux citoyens* (Paris: Herissant, 1760), 387–8.

[44]   George-Louis Leclerc, comte de Buffon, *Histoire naturelle, générale et particulière*, 36 vols (Paris: Imprimerie Royale, 1749–1788), II:489.

[45]   Rousseau, *Emile*, note to 495.

[46]   Pomme, *Essai sur les Affections vaporeuses*, 28.

Lignac is more nuanced in his portrayal of the relative degeneration of country and city dwellers. He sets up a fascinating fictional scenario: that of an individual transported from the empty "deserts" of Africa to the continent of Europe. This African is said to be at first mightily impressed by the industry of the agricultural workers and astonished by the energy of the "innumerable" inhabitants of the big cities, be it in search of money or pleasure. But the good opinion that he has developed of these people will evaporate, we are told, to the extent that he is able to look beyond the species and consider the individual. Our observer will see in the countryside men whom nature made robust, but who are degenerating insensibly. The inhabitants of the big cities will seem to his eyes to be unfortunate beings, on whom nature casts a tender gaze from time to time, but who do not notice her attentions. Those young men who leave the cities to fight (primarily the nobles, no doubt) are viewed as "effeminate creatures, already old in the springtime of their lives," the victims of "infirmities caused by love" (*On Man and Woman*, I:3–4).

Nevertheless, the relative health of country-dwelling youth, and especially the attribution of delayed puberty in the countryside to a lack of licentious influences— making this timing "natural" rather than artificial—is by far the dominant line taken in these treatises. There seem to be two countrysides, that of rural abundance and that of neglect, overwork, and want, each evoked to prove, essentially, the same point: if adequate food and moderate exercise are provided to young people and they are protected from lascivious influences, they will bloom both physically and morally. The urban poor get short shrift in most of these works, although Daignan adds "urban poverty" to his list of the causes of "this degeneration, or this impoverishment of the human species." He claims to base his observations on many years of studying young people "of all estates, all conditions, all countries, and consequently of all climates and constitutions" (I:vi), and notes that the "poverty of the common people living in the city" can be as nefarious as that of the country poor (I:viii). He worries also, that is, over those "country children" who do not enjoy the bounty he imagines for most, and in whom puberty is unnaturally delayed by physical, rather than moral causes, describing them, pitiably, as "malnourished, badly dressed, neglected, and forced to work very hard" (I:67). Daignan's Catholicity of interests reflects a change traced by Sean Quinlan in the targets of the social hygienists over the years (Daignan's *Tableau* appeared in 1786). Quinlan notes that while upper-class women dominate in the 1770s, attention is already shifting during that decade to the urban and the rural poor.[47]

The philosophical context of this urban–rural divide as it plays out in these treatises is of more interest in the context of this study than the sociological ramifications. Roussel enters most profoundly into the original causes of the deviation from "natural" physiology, putting forward the Rousseauian argument that our perfectibility leads us astray, whereas the lesser animals are protected from harm: "Reason and will detach man from the great chain that links all other beings; and the imperceptible strings that attach him to it still, are lax enough

---

47   Quinlan, *The Great Nation in Decline*, 54.

to permit him to distance himself a bit at times from the exact and straight path that the others are obligated to follow" (305). In yet another nod to Rousseau, Roussel attribute woman's "greater usefulness to society" (relative to men) to their greater "natural pity," an emotion he describes as "the basis for all social virtues" (32). In the most complementary fashion, women are thus viewed as adding an inestimable sympathy and grace to civilized gatherings, while men, incapable of such charm, dream up the technical and philosophical advances that make European civilization possible.

That the overall tone of the works by these physiologists is nevertheless one of despair illustrates the general assumption during the 1760s and 1770s that the price paid by the Europeans in adapting themselves to civilization in its highest form is ultimately too high to offset the loss of natural sanguinity and innocence. It is only as the Revolution approaches that the relative optimism of writers such as Bressy, carried high on the wave of Revolutionary reform, begins to dominate. But as the simultaneous presence of encomia to the benefits of advanced human social structures illustrates, the tension between nature and culture is ultimately left unresolved in these works, early or late. The implication is clear, however: the most glorious human beings, be they beautiful women or intellectually gifted (yet still adequately virile) men, are produced in an urban setting in which they have been carefully protected from the full influence of their culture until their adult temperaments have been fixed. Lise remains a comic figure, alongside her blushing, more virtuous, and equally ignorant country sisters. The prototypical country girl described in these treatises, who engages in plenty of physical activity, eats only healthy, locally produced food, and enjoys a moderate-to-light menstrual flow—that beauty destined for the downy-cheeked Adonis mentioned above—is the heroine neither of the novels, nor of the physiological treatises that I am examining. The urban ingénue described in the first part of this chapter is the star, and she is the product of the very city life attacked so vehemently by the physiologists. Her protective innocence is a hard won and thus all the more precious commodity, rather than the mere result of geographical coincidence.

Even Rousseau, as I go on to describe in the following chapter, does not make a heroine of one of his beloved alpine inhabitants, the *Valaisanes*. His Julie is a liminal character, raised as his subtitle tells us in "the foothills of the Alps," and thus midway between absolute purity and urban corruption. He also, famously, bemoans the "need" to write and publish his novel, in the preface to which he explains to his reader that he would rather have thrown the manuscript in the fire. As this overwrought claim illustrates, and while I will be demonstrating in the following chapters the importance of physiologically inflected themes in the novels of this period, the extent to which the novel as a genre is implicated in the decline pointed to by the physiologists is striking. Attacks against fiction by the era's moralists, centering primarily on the rise of the novel, have been explored from a historical perspective by Georges May, most influentially, but it is the connection between physiology and novel reading that most interests me.[48]

That the novel is in many ways a big city phenomenon accounts in great part for the link made by the physiologists between novel reading and moral degradation. So attractively evil are these works, at least in the eighteenth-century cultural imagination, that the writers of the hygiene treatises envision city girls eagerly partaking of their poison, unless most carefully supervised. This genre would seem to contain a substance capable of perverting the very essence of even the most innocent, prepubescent, sanguine country girl, otherwise destined to enjoy a moderate menstrual flow beginning at a relatively late age, and to be quite unbothered by whitish discharges, uterine spasms, strange quirks in appetite, and the urge to proposition strange men.

While in general the effects of novel reading on the brain are explored in these treatises in the most mechanical, deterministic of fashions—that is, the premature awakening of sexual desire prompts premature puberty and its attendant moral and physical ills—some physiologists, most notably Lignac, address the negative effects of novel reading in a more modern, psychological manner. Lignac informs us that men of letters are not the only individuals who avoid marriage, however much Tissot and others may have associated them with this unnatural suppression of the sexual function. There is another group, Lignac tells us, sexed female, and "larger than one might imagine," whose celibacy is adversely affecting the French population levels: "That is, the class of persons whose ardent imagination leads them to the continual reading [of novels]" (II:48). He declares that the number of such works has increased dramatically over the last one hundred years, and that this easy availability has created a generation of women who live in a thrill-seeking dream world. These are not Roussel's overly erudite bluestockings, whose "excremental" state prevents them from normal sexual functions (102–3); Lignac is pointing to otherwise healthy young women who waste their finest years looking for an impossibly perfect love, a relationship modeled on the unreal expectations they have acquired from novels (II:49; Roussel does make a similar point in a note to his *Physical and Moral System of Woman* in which he remarks that both the male and the female characters in novels possess "exaggerated moral and physical traits," 42, note a).

It is not at all coincidental that the novels under attack most often feature as heroines the very subset of the French population whose downfall they are said to be causing: young urban women in the prime of their brief careers as ingénues. The novelists are of course quite aware that this social group is assumed to be the most endangered by novel reading, as is clear in many tongue-in-cheek references in the works' prefaces. Whether serious or not, Rousseau declares in the preface to *The New Heloise* that he has given his work a title so unequivocal as to frighten off any worthy young woman. He adds, in a nod to the physiological consequences of

---

[48]   Georges May, *Le Dilemme du roman au XVIIIe siècle: Etude sur les rapports du roman et de la critique, 1715–1761* (Paris: Presses Universitaires de France, 1963).

novel reading that mimics the dramatic moment of defloration: "She who, in spite of this title, dares to read a single page is a ruined girl ... As she has started, let her finish reading: she has nothing more to lose."[49] It is this very vulnerability, of course, that makes young, newly postpubescent girls so attractive to the novelists, for such characters provide, in their unlimited capacity for seduction, both a clear tragic potential and a high titillation factor.

If the ingénues of the novels and the physiological treatises were only capable of high-level thinking—and we are assured that they are not—these young women might console themselves with the thought that both their innocence and their dangerous attractiveness will be short-lived. Once "nature's vow is fulfilled," the ingénue loses not only her virginity, but also her striking beauty, and the downhill slide is rapid, as Roussel describes in prime vitalist mode: "The expansive force, from which her organs took their color and their seductive form, diminishes, slows down; and a disagreeable flaccidity succeeds the supple and elastic firmness they once possessed, if the weight gain that adulthood normally brings on does not support them" (83). That older women are particularly pitiable in their reaction to the loss of their "elastic firmness" is a frequent commonplace of both the medical and the fictional texts of this period. Roussel describes the typical aging woman who seeks desperately to hold on to her waning beauty as follows: "There is a period of time, too short no doubt, when she is able attract men with the remaining charms that recall those she no longer possesses. She redoubles her efforts to preserve these precious, useless leftovers" (84–5).

In exploring the eighteenth-century literary archetype of the ingénue in the next chapters of this study, I focus on the extent to which the highly determined female physiological specimens presented in these fictional works break from the limits placed on their sisters as described in the physiological texts, usually with great difficulty. Perhaps the most fascinating, and certainly the most influential of such heroines, is the subject of my next chapter: the paradigmatic Julie d'Etange, created by the same theorist who brought to life *Emile*'s Sophie. I argue that although these two fictional creations have been cited as representing a highly contradictory view of womanhood, there is no real contradiction in Rousseau's having produced these two seemingly disparate visions of womanhood, for Julie is just as firmly rooted in the material, deterministic world described in *Emile* as is her ideological sister, Sophie.

---

[49]   Jean-Jacques Rousseau, *Julie ou La Nouvelle Héloïse*, in *Oeuvres complètes*, II:6.

Chapter 3
Julie d'Etange, or Sexuality and the Virtuous Heroine

> Although [medicine] furnishes M. Rousseau with the very arms he uses
> to combat it, at times this philosopher's ideas take on the strong colors that
> scientific truths always lend to eloquence.
> —Pierre Roussel, *The Moral and Physical System of Woman*

The vitalists' opinion of Jean-Jacques Rousseau was somewhat mixed. Elizabeth A. Williams notes that Théophile de Bordeu treated Rousseau with "irony and more than a measure of condescension," but later vitalists were more impressed by Rousseau's success in reaching a popular audience.[1] He was considered part of a loose community of authors writing for the public good, especially with works such as *Emile* and the *Discourse on Inequality* in which the dangers of the civilized state are so vividly painted. Rousseau's lack of formal medical training made his incursions into physiology a bit suspect however, not to mention his frequent and passionate attacks on the medical profession. He dismissed the vast majority of medical practitioners as charlatans, praising only those doctors who were willing to acknowledge that they knew little to nothing about how the body functioned.[2] These attacks would culminate in an accusation in Book Eleven of the *Confessions* that the eminent Bordeu himself had starved a young patient to death in the blind pursuit of a cure.[3]

Roussel nevertheless exaggerates when he declares in the epigraph above that Rousseau "combats medicine" in his writings, for the author of *Emile* was an avid proponent of hygiene theory, that branch of medicine central to the vitalist agenda. In Book IX of the *Confessions* we learn that Rousseau had even planned to write a work explicitly devoted to hygiene, to be called *Sensitive Morality, or The Wise Man's Materialism*, in which he would have taught his readers how to control their affective states by carefully managing their exposure to various external stimuli,

---

[1] Elizabeth A. Williams, *A Cultural History of Medical Vitalism in Enlightenment Montpellier* (Aldershot, UK and Burlington, VT: Ashgate, 2003), 224.

[2] Rousseau writes in a letter of 19 October 1761: "Far from trying to die, it was to continue to live until the last possible moment that I gave up on the ruses of doctors. Twenty years of torments and experiments have been sufficient to teach me the nature of my illness and the insufficiency of their art" (*Correspondance complète de Jean-Jacques Rousseau*, ed. R.A. Leigh, 52 vols [Oxford: The Voltaire Foundation, 1965–1998], IX:188).

[3] Jean-Jacques Rousseau, *Confessions*, in *Oeuvres complètes*, 4 vols. (Paris: Gallimard, 1959–1969), I:550.

including "climate, the seasons, sounds, colors, darkness, light, the elements, food, noise, silence, movement, [and] repose."[4]

Instead of writing this how-to book, Rousseau tells us, he fell into a reverie and began drafting "letters" to and from an imaginary woman, impassioned missives that would become the best-selling novel of the eighteenth century: *Julie or The New Heloise* (1761).[5] Rousseau explains in the *Confessions* that the fantasizing behind this novel was occasioned by the lack of any flesh-and-blood woman who came close to his feminine ideal—a harsh indictment of French women in general and more particularly of Thérèse Levasseur, his live-in partner and mother to his five (abandoned) children. But while the oneiric and fantastical birth of Julie d'Etange would seem to point to a thoroughly ethereal character, I argue in this chapter that Rousseau's heroine was quite bound to her body and that an appreciation of the intensity of this physico-moral connection is crucial to our understanding of this novel.[6] Jean Ehrard is one of the few scholars to have taken an interest in the materialist ethos of the work, arguing that to do otherwise is to misread it: "It is thus to misinterpret Rousseau's novel, and probably to block any comprehension of its immense success, to see it, from some 'pre-Romantic' perspective, as only the novel of 'sensitive souls.'"[7]

In placing *The New Heloise* in the context of the reinvention of femaleness and female sexuality in the mid-eighteenth century, I follow Ehrard's lead. In the first part of this chapter, I consider the many details Rousseau provides concerning Julie's body, including the size, color, and consistency of her "perfect" young breasts, her reactions to sexual stimuli, and the causes and effects of her illnesses. These physical details are to be understood as outward indicators of Julie's inherent mental qualities, for the novel attributes the existence of this paragon of femininity above all to geographical location. Her extraordinary *sensibilité* may mark her as an exception among women, but this innate quality is also to be understood, in great part, as a product of her environment. Whether an "accident" of nature or a divine gift, this heightened ability to feel would never have blossomed into an exquisite moral sensibility had our heroine been born in Paris—something of a moot point, of course, for such a birth would have had to be truly a miraculous occurrence, by the logic of Rousseau's novel.

---

[4]   Rousseau, *Confessions*, 408.

    [5]   On the success of Rousseau's novel, see Anna Attridge, "The Reception of *La Nouvelle Héloïse*," *Studies on Voltaire and the Eighteenth Century* 120 (1974): 227–67; Claude Labrosse, *Lire au XVIIIe siècle*: La Nouvelle Héloïse *et ses lecteurs* (Lyons: Presses Universitaires de Lyons, 1985); and Raymond Birn, *Forging Rousseau: Print, commerce, and cultural manipulation in the late Enlightenment* (Oxford: SVEC, 2001:8).

    [6]   This chapter expands on an argument I have made in "Julie's Breasts, Julie's Scars: Physiology and Character in *La Nouvelle Héloïse*," *Studies in Eighteenth-Century Culture* 36 (March 2007): 1–20.

    [7]   Jean Ehrard, "Le Corps de Julie," in *Thèmes et figures du siècle des Lumières*, ed. Raymond Trousson (Geneva: Droz, 1980), 101.

As I argue in the second part of this chapter, the emphasis on determinism in *The New Heloise* is only half the story of this novel's "immense success." The physiological elements ("scientific truths," in Roussel's terms) that are so clearly present in this work do not account for the popularity of what is above all a masterpiece of fiction writing ("eloquence"). Julie is no simple country girl whose emotional life follows an equally simple path, for such a character would have been of little interest to the reading public. She is instead liminal in both her geographical placement and her social standing. She is a physiological mean of femininity whose parents raise her in a relatively protected manner, but these same, imperfect parents also create the circumstances in which her tragic love affair with Saint-Preux will take place. Julie's mother begins the process by hiring Saint-Preux to tutor Julie while her father is away, allowing her love for this young man to blossom. Upon her father's return, this proud man seals his daughter's fate by insisting that Saint-Preux does not possess the social standing necessary to marry a d'Etange and that Julie must instead marry the much older Wolmar.

After following the course of Julie's love affair with Saint-Preux and the suppression of her feelings for her lover following her marriage, I consider how her exemplary death allows Rousseau to reconcile the two distinct parts into which he divides his novel: the story of Julie's youthful affair and the description of her married life at Clarens. These two parts are equivalent to two paths, those of nature versus civilization. Julie is forced to make an impossible choice as the first part of the novel ends. Listening to the "voice of nature" would mean eloping with her lover and thus abandoning, even perhaps literally killing, her parents. Acceding to the demands of culture and marrying her father's friend Wolmar would mean sacrificing not only her own happiness but also the happiness and perhaps even the life of Saint-Preux. She of course chooses the latter path, but I argue that the physiological manifestations of this choice are many and highly significant. As the novel ends, Julie's quasi-suicidal leap into the water to save her child and the lingering death that follows allow Rousseau to explore at length how the addition of a transcendent, immortal soul to his era's deterministic vision of the mind–body connection allows his heroine to reconcile, finally, these two competing and contradictory aspects of her earth-bound virtue.

Rousseau's novel was extraordinarily popular among women intellectuals, including the memorialist I examine in my final chapter, Marie-Jeanne Roland. The devotion of such women to Rousseau's work has often been seen as problematic, given the reputation for misogyny attached to his writings even in his own day, and especially to "Sophie, or Woman" (the last section of *Emile*), in which he attacks educated or even excessively clever women.[8] That Julie's successful engagement with love, duty, faith, and fidelity was apparently quite attractive to

---

8   Jean-Jacques Rousseau, *Emile, ou de l'éducation*, in *Oeuvres complètes*, IV:736. The contrast between Julie and Sophie generated considerable critical commentary, in Rousseau's own day and in our own. See Gita May, "Rousseau's 'Antifeminism' Reconsidered," and Vera Lee, "The Edifying Examples," both in *French Women and the Age of Enlightenment*, ed. Samia I. Spencer (Bloomington: Indiana University Press, 1984), 309–17, 345–54.

such unlikely readers—unlikely, of course, judged by our current standards—makes an examination of her virtue in the context of the era's physiological theories of femininity all the more telling. The circumstances of Julie's death are particularly significant in this regard, and after exploring the striking conclusion to the novel, I end the present chapter with a consideration of how two well-known and highly successful women novelists, Marie-Jeanne Riccoboni and Isabelle de Charrière, end their own works in which women are faced with similar impossible situations. These women authors create significantly different solutions for their own virtuous heroines, I argue, solutions in which the physiological determinism present in Rousseau's novel plays no role.

Rousseau's Materialized Dream Woman

Julie's childhood and her passage through the tumultuous revolution of puberty precede the opening of this tale of thwarted love, but are implicit in that as the novel begins we meet a heroine who is clearly the ideal postpubescent female specimen. In the full bloom of young adulthood, Julie d'Etange is primed, in other words, for marriage (sex) with a suitable partner, and has indeed already found that partner in the adoring Saint-Preux, whose first lovesick letter to her opens the work. For while the novel's title may evoke the cliché role of the seducing tutor, Saint-Preux's obvious suitability as the object of Julie's desire makes him a "natural" choice for her, in the full sense of that adjective, with her father's opposition to their marriage to be understood as placing him in the category of the "bad parent" of the hygiene treatises. He is more solicitous of his own misplaced pride in social status than of his daughter's health and happiness. In this novel, in other words, the standard tale of love thwarted by parental authority takes on a much larger social argument, reflecting the medical revolution currently under way as well as the changing image of female sexual virtue at the heart of this new theoretical view of sexuality. As a fictional character, Julie may overcome the limitations placed on the young women in the physiological treatises (Sophie included), but she is subject to the same forces and must struggle mightily to maintain her own virtue in a corrupt society, and despite succumbing to a premarital sexual affair.

Saint-Preux's letters provide much of the evidence I will be citing in tracing the consequences of this corruption on this inherently perfect young woman, for her lover is of necessity a fascinated observer of Julie's physical and moral states. Julie's letters to Saint-Preux and to her devoted friend Claire are an important source of information as well, for Julie is an unusually attentive and intelligent analyst of her own emotional reactions. She is also far more concerned with social mores and virtue in general than is Saint-Preux, in keeping with Rousseau's views on the passive manifestation of virtue in women and the courageous action expected of virtuous men. Most importantly, Julie seeks to capitalize on what she learns in order to improve her moral being over time, while Saint-Preux is for the most part content to nourish his despair (when he is not plotting to free Julie of her social chains). The first part of this novel, in which we read of the lovers' affair, thus represents something of a "natural" conduct manual for young women trapped in impossible situations, conveying information that is experience based and thus more intuitive than learned. The second part of the work, in which we witness Julie's married life at Clarens under the direction of her eminently reasonable husband Wolmar, provides a more formal lesson in how to live in the context of (and to a great extent in spite of) one's culture, along the lines of the hygiene manual Rousseau set out to write before "Julie" captured his imagination.

That climate plays a major role in Julie's development into the young woman we meet as the novel opens is indicated in the work's subtitle: "The Letters of Two Lovers Living in a Small Village at the Foot of the Alps."[9] The strongest statement as to the meaning of Julie's physical provenance is found in letter 23, written by Saint-Preux to Julie. This missive is among the work's best known in that it is a defense of the Valais, that isolated and elevated Swiss region that had been recently mocked in the article "Cretin" of the *Encyclopédie* (1754) by none other than Diderot's co-editor, the eminent mathematician Jean le Rond d'Alembert. The distance between the two lovers that creates the need for the letter is strategic, for Saint-Preux has left the "foot of the Alps" at Julie's request. Her father is returning home after the eight-month absence that had enabled their love to develop, and she hopes to convince him to consider the lesser-born Saint-Preux as a possible son-in-law. Monsieur d'Etange is also retiring from a long military career, and will soon be a fixture in the house and in Julie's life, a not insignificant change to relations between the lovers.

Heartsick at the separation, Saint-Preux climbs ever higher into the Swiss mountains, where he finds solace not in "Romantic" solitude but rather in the mountain atmosphere. He writes to his beloved that the "pure and subtle" air he breathes is working to moderate his passions and calm his frenzied mind: "I doubt that any violent agitation, any vaporous malady, would last during a prolonged stay here, and I am surprised that a bath in the salutary and beneficent mountain air is not one of the principal remedies of both medicine and morality."[10] He goes on to describe the inhabitants of the Valais, those beings who have bathed in this "salutary" atmosphere since birth. He is particularly struck by the beauty of the women, possessed of the most stunning complexions. One aspect of their bodies bothers him quite a bit, however: the "enormous amplitude" of their breasts. Saint-Preux qualifies his reaction to these attributes as one of "shock," indicating that such exaggerated displays of femininity make him somewhat uncomfortable and go against his esthetic ideal.

---

[9]   For the history and significance of Rousseau's changing titles, see Philip Stewart, "Half-Title, or *Julie* Beheaded" (*Romanic Review* 86 [1995]: 36–43).

[10]   Jean-Jacques Rousseau, *Julie, ou La Nouvelle Héloïse*, in *Oeuvres complètes*, II:78. Future references in the text.

The relationship between breast size and beauty that Saint-Preux observes will make its way as "evidence" into Moreau de la Sarthe's *Natural History of Woman*, in which this passage from the *New Heloise* is cited to strengthen the claim that in those European regions with the highest elevation, and principally in Switzerland, "the male form generally develops beautifully; but women's bodies are exaggerated in a manner that makes them more pleasing and voluptuous than truly beautiful."[11] Saint-Preux's own development of his physical observations follows the scientific findings of his day, for he makes the connection between the physical and the moral realm in declaring that these women of the high Alps exhibit an equally unbalanced sense of shame. One word from Saint-Preux suffices to make the women of the Valais blush uncontrollably, he tells Julie, and while this heightened color increases the beauty of their complexion, such intense modesty also renders ordinary conversation impossible. Saint-Preux tells Julie that during meals, even judges' wives remain standing, "like servants."

The city-dwelling opposites of these overly modest women are described by Saint-Preux in letter II.21, written during his visit to that capital of decadence, Paris. While Saint-Preux finds the female inhabitants of this urban cesspool, as it is so often portrayed, too skinny overall, he is particularly displeased with their chests, which he describes as at "the other extremity of the *Valaisanes*" (266). He declares the breasts of Parisian women to be not only overly small but also of only "mediocre whiteness," failings apparently attributable to the pressures of licentious city life. The relationship between breast size and modesty is wonderfully expressed in Saint-Preux's declaration that no good man faced with the "self-assured gaze" of a *Parisienne* could prevent himself from lowering his eyes—at which point he would be faced with an illusion: "With tightly laced corsets they try to impose consistency; there are other ways of imposing color" (266).

We are not surprised to learn, two letters later, that Julie is the perfect medium between these two extremes. Saint-Preux tells her that only in their "blinding whiteness" do the overlarge attractions of the women of the Valais match her own. As for size, Julie's breasts are perfection itself (he evokes the famous drinking cup molded from a breast of Helen of Troy). Morally as well Julie represents an ideal mean, for she is able to converse easily in the presence of men, provided that the topics and the situation are appropriate. As the geographic and cultural determiners of chest size in this novel teach us, Julie's perfect chest is far more than a figurative metonymy of her feminine virtue. Her breasts are to be understood as actual fleshy embodiments of that virtue. The importance of the size of Julie's breasts is best illustrated by a correction Rousseau ordered made to one of the plates prepared for his novel. He wrote to the artist, a young Genevan named François Coindet: "I find that in all the drawings Julie and Claire are too flat chested. Swiss women

---

[11]   Louis-Jacques Moreau de la Sarthe, *Histoire naturelle de la femme*, 3 vols (Paris: Duprat, Letellier, 1803), I:351.

are not that way. Monsieur Coindet is no doubt aware that the women of our country have larger breasts than Parisian women."[12]

That this correction had more than merely esthetic importance is highlighted by our knowledge that, aside from her highly significant breasts, Julie is not otherwise a strikingly beautiful physical specimen. Rousseau is concerned with accuracy of representation, not with enhancing the charms of his heroine. Jean Ehrard points out that Julie is allowed subtle faults that previous female characters would never have exhibited: traces of veins visible on her skin, a small scar on her lip. While the presence of visible veins, as we have seen in the previous chapter, may be yet another reference to her physiological perfection, rather than a "fault," Ehrard is certainly right about the scar, and more importantly, even Julie's lover does not believe her to be the "most beautiful" of women, judged objectively. Saint-Preux writes of the jealousy he feels at seeing the men at a gathering irresistibly attracted to Julie, despite the presence, he tells her, of women "more beautiful" than she is.

From a purely physical point of view, Julie's body is to be understood as an irresistible mean of femininity, down to the size of her breasts. She is identical in this sense to Sophie, Emile's intended, of whom we are told: "Sophie is not beautiful, but when they are near her men forget beautiful women, and beautiful women are unhappy with themselves."[13] Rather than an extreme of feminine charm, Sophie is like Julie to be understood as all the more desirable in that she represents an absolute norm of femininity. In the same way, although with the addition of an all-important spiritual transcendence appropriate to her fictional rather than pedagogical function, Julie's "perfection" lies in her unusual conformity to a standard of femininity.

Rousseau does not present the simplest of lifestyles as the most appealing in *The Nouvelle Heloise*, any more than he accepts any physical extreme as the most appealing. The inhabitants of the Valais do not, in other words, represent a moral ideal any more than they are to be taken as a physical archetype, however much Rousseau may seek to defend them from their attackers. The calm that Saint-Preux experiences in the higher elevations is somehow "unnatural," not fully human in its excessiveness, just like the "blushing virtue" and physical charms of the *Valaisanes*. These high mountains would never produce a proper mate for Emile, nor are they a suitable setting for the characters of a morally uplifting novel. We are to understand that had Julie been born high in the mountains, the damage to her moral complexity would have been greater than the distortion to her chest. Living in the foothills of the Alps, she is close enough to benefit from their pure air, but not so close that her well-modulated modesty devolves into uncontrollable blushing. Had she been

---

[12]   Letter of 5 November 1760, *Correspondance complète*, VII:295. In a passage from the *Confessions* often cited alongside this letter, Rousseau is a bit more vulgar: "Neither my heart nor my senses would ever be capable of seeing a woman in someone with no breasts" (412). For more on the breast in Rousseau's work, see Sue Wiseman, "From the Luxurious Breast to the Virtuous Breast: The Body Politic Transformed," *Textual Practice* 11:3 (1997): 477–92.

[13]   Rousseau, *Emile*, 746.

a *Valaisanne*, it would have been impossible for the passion between herself and Saint-Preux to develop and take hold; impossible for her father to have developed an exaggerated notion of noble birth; and most important, impossible for Julie to triumph over the resulting pain through self-sacrifice, and for this triumph to symbolize the mysterious manner in which she transcends the limitations of her sex.

We are informed early on of this innate superiority, as I will briefly consider here before moving on to explore several key moments in Julie's life that demonstrate how tightly her morality is physically grounded by the deterministic rules of her era. Julie's character is established to a great degree by contrast with her friend Claire, a delightful, attractive young woman of standard morals and intelligence, who is predictably in awe of her friend. It is Claire and several other secondary characters, rather than the amorous Saint-Preux, who best express the mystery of Julie's magnetic attraction. Claire writes to her friend:

> We both love virtue; honesty is equally dear to us; our talents are the same; I have almost as much wit as you do, and am scarcely less pretty. I know all of that quite well; and in spite of it all you dominate me, you subjugate me, you confound me, your spirit crushes my own, and I am nothing before you … Explain this enigma, if you can; as for me, I understand nothing of it. (409)

The explanation has already been given to the reader by Milord Edouard, that British connoisseur of women who immediately recognizes the quality of his friend Saint-Preux's love object: "There is only one Julie" (198).

Ehrard writes of this passage: "As an experienced man, Edouard discerns in [Julie's] beauty the inalterable presence of the 'common model'—the first model, Diderot's 'ideal model'—from which ordinary persons always diverge."[14] Chance has intervened, however atavistically, to make Julie "exquisitely," "uniquely" normal in her physico-moral configuration. Rousseau is in other words no proponent of the Lockean tabula rasa, but rather embraces the theory of innate temperament so common in his era and so dear in particular to the vitalists. Daniel Mornet notes that in the margins of Rousseau's copy of *On Mind* (1758), he disputes Helvétius's statement that all minds are equal at birth and subsequently formed by education: "If he claims that education is all important he must also prove that it causes differences in temperament, skin color, stature, for all these are the end result of a chain of causes that we do not clearly comprehend."[15] Saint-Preux echoes this view in letter V.3, on the topic of the proper education of children (he is quoting Julie): "In addition to the constitution of the species as a whole, each person is born with a particular temperament that determines his individual genius and his character, and that one must neither change nor constrain, but rather form and perfect" (563).

---

[14]   Ehrard, "Le Corps de Julie," 99.

[15]   Daniel Mornet, *Les Sciences de la nature en France au XVIIIᵉ siècle: Un Chapitre de l'histoire des idées* (Paris: Armand Colin, 1911), 65, note 1.

The cultural setting in which she has been raised has exposed Julie to some of the pressures said to cause distortion in "ordinary persons," including (mildly) licentious conversations with Claire's governess (43). We are nevertheless to understand that unlike Claire, Julie has resisted such influences and is possessed of an unshakeable, innate sense of virtue. It is the circumstance in which she finds herself with regard to Saint-Preux, not her own moral compass, that is out of balance. Most importantly, we are not to think that Julie's physical affair with Saint-Preux is in any way a contradiction of her transcendent morality. Readers are to accept that Rousseau's heroine makes that fundamental eighteenth-century transition from virgin to sexually active woman outside of marriage, yet retains her reputation for virtuous perfection.

Not all readers, needless to say, accepted this argument. Voltaire—quick as always to ridicule an author he regarded as one of the enemies of social enlightenment—quite thoroughly mocks this aspect of the novel in his *Letters on The New Heloise* (1761). He even attributes a coarse and scabrous statement to the newly married Wolmar, said to be "very pleased with the barrel although another had pierced it" (we learn late in the novel that Wolmar had been aware of the affair before he married Julie). In the same piece, Voltaire defends Parisian women against Saint-Preux's aspersions concerning their lack of beauty: "No; they are neither as skinny nor as weather beaten as you claim."[16]

There are of course, *pace* Voltaire, many extenuating factors working in favor of our acceptance of Julie's postlapsarian virtue. For example, despite the obvious injustice of her father's opposition to Saint-Preux, rejection of or rebellion against paternal dictates is not in the least involved in Julie's decision to consummate her relationship with Saint-Preux. She refuses to flee with him when faced with the impossibility of their ever marrying, fearing that this abandonment will kill her parents (her brother, their only other child, is dead). She soon comes to realize, however, that should she abandon Saint-Preux and marry according to her parents' wishes, she will be the cause of his death instead of their own. Her decision to have sex with this persistent lover outside of the sacrament of marriage is thus presented as a Christ-like move. Julie writes: "It was necessary to sacrifice those who gave me life, my lover, or myself. Without knowing what I was doing I chose my own misfortune; I forgot everything and thought only of love" (96, letter from Julie to Claire).

The intensity of Saint-Preux's suffering is indeed striking, for Julie describes him as "in convulsive fits, ready to faint at my feet." She retrospectively acknowledges some responsibility for the physical affair in that she allowed herself to witness these "fits": "I dared too much in contemplating this dangerous spectacle. I felt myself moved by his transports" (96). It is however Claire's intervention in writing to Saint-Preux and luring him back to Julie's side that ultimately brings the two lovers together. She does so, she insists, in order to save her friend's life, for Julie's belief that she would never again see Saint-Preux had given rise to a raging fever

---

[16] Voltaire, "*Lettres sur* La Nouvelle Héloïse," *Mélanges de Voltaire* (Paris: Gallimard, 1961), 404, 405.

of the most dangerous variety (*une fièvre ardente*). Fortunately, Claire understands that physical union with Saint-Preux is the prescribed cure (*le spécifique*) for Julie's sufferings and tells Saint-Preux that he must return. We note that the lives of both these lovers had to be at stake in order for them to consummate their affair—an overdetermined case of sacrificial copulation, presented with a clearly medicinal tone as the only possible life-saving cure for what ailed them.

In letter I.29, Julie admonishes Claire for acting as amateur physician while at the same time acknowledging the efficacity of the prescribed treatment: "What demon inspired you to summon him back, the cruel one who has dishonored me? Must his perfidious attentions have brought me back to life only to make life odious to me?" (95). In the following letter, Claire responds that Julie's loss of virtue was a price that Claire, at least, was willing to pay to avoid the loss of her friend: "I felt that [your] heart beating with love must either be happy or die; and when the fear of succumbing made you banish your lover with so many tears, I judged that either you would cease to exist, or he would soon be called back. But imagine my fear when I saw you no longer wishing to live, and so close to death! Do not blame your lover, or yourself, for a sin for which I bear the most guilt, because I foresaw it without preventing it" (97).

In a much later, retrospective letter to Saint-Preux (III.18), Julie concisely sums up the episode: "I saw you, I was cured, and I perished" (344). Adding a final patina of disculpation to the event is the overarching "naturalness" attached to the physical consummation of the strong moral union between Saint-Preux and Julie. As even her future husband will acknowledge in discussing Julie's past, one goes against nature by resisting true love. Such resistance is all the more unnatural when one is young, innately virtuous, and a paragon of sensibility. Saint-Preux states the matter clearly in the first letter of the novel: "We are so young that nothing has altered our natural inclinations" (32). This axiom is echoed by the Savoyard vicar of *Emile*, for as he relates his own youthful indiscretions, the vicar declares: "It is in vain that they forbid us this or that, we feel only faint remorse when doing what is permitted by a well-ordered nature, and even less when doing what nature prescribes."[17]

That our two young lovers are in the sway of this powerful natural law is evident from their first kiss. Nowhere in the novel is their sensibility so strikingly evoked as in the description of this embrace in the famous grove of trees (*bosquet*, letter I.14). Julie is so very sensitive, and so very unprepared for what she experiences, that the surprise of this intense physical contact causes her to swoon, but not, we are to note, to faint entirely. Rousseau is quite specific about this distinction in his description of the accompanying engraving: "Julie must swoon and not faint. The entire picture must breathe a voluptuous intoxication made even more touching by a certain air of modesty."[18] Saint-Preux's reaction to this first embrace is equally revealing. As the male to Julie's exemplary female, he is set on

---

[17]   Rousseau, *Emile*, 566.

[18]   Rousseau, *Sujets d'estampes*, in *Oeuvres complètes*, II:762.

fire, rather than incapacitated. He "reproaches" Julie for having planned this kiss as his reward for good behavior, for it has left him in a toxic state: "I am drunk, or rather mad. My senses are altered, all my faculties are troubled by this deadly kiss. You wanted to soothe my sufferings! Cruel woman! You made them more bitter. It was poison that I took from your lips" (63). He ends his letter by again emphasizing the "bitterness" of these poisonous embraces: "No keep your kisses, they are too much for me … they are too bitter, too penetrating; they pierce, they burn to the marrow" (65).

Voltaire seizes with obvious delight on Rousseau's use of the adjective "bitter" (*âcre*) to describe Julie's kisses: "Julie, in the presence of her cousin Claire, gives her master a very long and very *bitter* kiss about which he complains a great deal, and the next day the master fathers a child by his student."[19] But while Voltaire dismisses this choice of adjective as merely indicative of Rousseau's lack of sensitivity to the nuances of the French language, the more attentive (or perhaps the less negatively motivated reader) observes that the link between bitterness and sensuality is emphasized elsewhere in the novel. When Saint-Preux extols the quality of the mountain air of the Valais, going so far as to recommend "air baths" for those suffering from the vapors, he notes the absence of "bitterness" in the tranquility one enjoys at these heights: "One's reflections take on some sort of great and sublime character, in proportion to the objects that draw one's attention, some sort of tranquil voluptuousness that has nothing bitter nor sensual" (78–9). The physical suffering of the lovers as they first embrace is thus geographically determined, for Julie and Saint-Preux are removed from this calm mountain atmosphere. They live out their love in a world of denser air and more complex human interactions, making geographical location, as always, one important source of the painful intensity of their passion.

That the slings and arrows of love are made literal by Rousseau is very much in keeping with the emphasis in this novel on the interrelationship between the physical and the moral realms. Voltaire's attack on Rousseau's "bitter kisses" becomes, in this context, as symptomatically oversophisticated as the reaction of the Parisian of whom Saint-Preux inquires how it is possible for ex-lovers to meet without experiencing severe physical symptoms. His Parisian interlocutor cuts off Saint-Preux's provincial query with a curt, mocking reply: "You make me laugh, he interrupted, with your shudderings! You would thus have our women do nothing other than fall into faints?" (272). The insouciance of Parisian lovers, the reader is to understand, is not the result of sophistication, but is rather a symptom of their lack of emotional attachment, born of the tepid, "merely" pleasurable physical passion they experience. In sharp contrast, Saint-Preux literally burns when he first kisses his ideal woman, while Julie's half-faints represent the feminine version of the intensity of feeling a mere kiss can evoke in the inhabitants of the countryside.

---

[19]   Voltaire, *Lettres sur* La Nouvelle Héloïse, 400.

This half-faint also plays a significant symbolic role in that it allows Julie to retain a claim to modesty while simultaneously exhibiting her capacity for intense pleasure. We are told in letter V.2 that Julie "has a soul and body equally sensitive" (541), but any fictional eighteenth-century woman with the least claim to virtue must be construed as biologically programmed not to seek out sexual pleasure. To do otherwise is to act like an unnatural woman, "a monster" like Laclos's Merteuil, whose active sexual appetite and materialist worldview I explore in the following chapter. Julie becomes the mouthpiece for this essential Rousseauian dictum on female virtue when she writes, in an echo of Book Five of *Emile*: "Attack and defense, men's audacity, women's modesty, are not only conventions, as the philosophes believe, but natural institutions easily explained, and from which one easily deduces all the other moral distinctions [between the sexes]" (128).

In the analysis of how true love operates that follows, Julie uses a chemical analogy to describe the process by which the "divine fire" with which lovers burn spiritualizes physical desire at the same time that it ensures mutual fidelity: "It seems to me that true love is the most chaste of unions. It is true love, it is its divine fire, which is able to purify our natural inclinations, and concentrate them in one object" (138). She is writing this letter (I.50) primarily to chastise Saint-Preux for some rather forward language that he had used with her at a gathering (he had been drinking). She accuses him of having lost respect for her, now that they have made love. True lovers, she states, never use "the coarse language" of debauchery. Rather than merely acting on physical desire, they discreetly *employ* it, in order to increase the constancy of their love: "They do not desire, they love. The heart does not follow the senses, it guides them; it covers over their excesses with a delicious veil" (138). The intensity of sensual love misleads men, who seek out its "burning fire" as an end in itself. Such behavior may be necessary to the survival of the species, yet Julie insists that Saint-Preux recognize love as she sees it: "Sensual man, will you never learn to love? Remember, remember that sensation, so calm and sweet, that you once felt and that you described in such a touching and tender tone" (237).

The sensation that Saint-Preux had once felt was the result of the second and last time the two manage to arrange to make love. In letter I.55, Saint-Preux describes the calm that succeeded their lovemaking as having finally taught him the true meaning of happiness. Glossing quickly over the act itself ("the transports of the most ardent love ... those intoxicating favors"), he elaborates at length on the "pure, continuous, universal voluptuousness" of lying next to Julie, "your face against mine, your breath on my cheek, and your arm around my neck." Their postcoital kisses are far from "painful"; they are described rather as "those kisses that a languorous voluptuousness allowed us to savor slowly" (148). The calm quality of this scene is all the more striking in that the previous letter, written in Julie's *cabinet*, or dressing room, has just presented the reader with the high fever pitch of Saint-Preux's lust. As he waits to be admitted to the inner sanctum, he allows his gaze to caress the "breasts" of Julie's corset: "In front, two slight contours ... O spectacle of voluptuousness! ... the whalebone has ceded to the force of the impressions ... delicious imprints, I kiss you a thousand times! ... Gods! Gods!" It is at this climactic moment that Saint-Preux—still writing, of course—is painfully "penetrated" by Julie: "I breathe you in with the air that you breathed; you penetrate my substance; your presence is burning and painful for me!" (147). Whether we are to understand the source of this pain as Saint-Preux's frustration with the limits of his experience in the *cabinet*, or as the result of some bitter, burning quality possessed by the actual physical "traces" of Julie's presence, or more likely as a combination of both, it is clear that for this paradigmatically passionate male, calm voluptuousness can come only after the physical release of lovemaking.

That forces beyond their control drive these ideal lovers to consummate a relationship forbidden by their society reflects the contradictory position that love occupies in Rousseau's overall philosophy. The clearest expression of this ambiguity is found in the history of human civilization outlined in the *Discourse on Inequality*. That Rousseau never preached a return to his famous version of the "state of nature"—a common misreading of the *Discourse*—has been demonstrated by a number of commentators.[20] To the contrary, Rousseau would have our phylogenetic development frozen at the point when humans first gathered together in small, stationary tribal groups. The discontents of this early form of civilization do not yet outweigh the benefits, although the downside of continuous association with others of our species is said to include the birth of the passions. All violent emotions—all feelings other than pity—are quite absent from the calm mental life of Rousseau's originary solitary wanderers, including love. But while this last emotion is presented as in itself a welcome development of tribal life, it soon gives birth to a more insidious passion: "A sweet and tender sentiment insinuates itself into the soul, and at the least opposition becomes an impetuous furor: jealousy awakens with love; discord triumphs, and the gentlest of passions receives sacrifices of human blood."[21]

We have just been told that each "tribe" or nation is unified not by laws (there is no social contract per se at this point), but rather by sharing "the same type of life and food, and by the influence of climate." This climatic determination of emotional intensity would seem to hold true in *The New Heloise* as well, for Parisians are said to be, as described above, quite tepid lovers, for whom jealousy is a laughable weakness. In the Valais, any intense physical attraction would be attenuated by the thin mountain air, and lack of contact between the sexes makes Valaisan jealousy a moot point. A letter to Saint-Preux from Milord Edouard confirms that we are to read this contrast between the high Alps and the urban environment of Paris as a lesson in comparative anthropology: "Your first observations were of simple people, almost fresh from the hands of nature, as if

---

[20] See especially Jonathan Marks, *Perfection and Disharmony in the Thought of Jean-Jacques Rousseau* (Cambridge: Cambridge University Press, 2005).

[21] Rousseau, *Discours sur l'origine et les fondements de l'inégalité parmi les hommes*, in *Oeuvres complètes*, III:169.

to serve as a comparison. Exiled in the capital of the most celebrated people of the universe, you then leapt, one might say, to the other extremity: your mind may extrapolate the intermediary stages" (524). As for the inhabitants of the foothills of the Alps, we are back to a version of the intense jealousy felt by the originary tribal dwellers, for Saint-Preux, true to his intermediary character, experiences a degree of jealousy equal to the burning passion he feels for Julie. When he challenges Milord Edouard to a duel for innocently admiring Julie, unaware that she and Saint-Preux are lovers, it becomes clear that this area of Europe is the closest one gets, in the corrupted "modern" world, to the ideal stage of human development Rousseau had earlier described in his *Discourse.*

The promptness with which Julie becomes pregnant also indicates to readers that these two lovers are the favored children of an ideal natural love in an ideal setting. She hints at the possibility of a child soon after their first physical union, although at this point she has no reason to believe herself pregnant, only a desire to be so: "Ah! if from my sins might be born the way to repair them!" (105). Physiologically, she has every reason to be hopeful, according to the theories of her day. The belief that a woman could only conceive if she gave herself willingly (and thus excreted female "semen") had been promoted for centuries. Pierre Roussel's description of the process postdates the novel but merits a long quotation both for the detail he provides and for his poetic enthusiasm:

> Everyone seems to agree that conception is more certain when the two individuals involved lose themselves at the same time in the transports of which it is the fruit. This short alienation in which their souls seem for a moment to pass entirely into the new being that results, and the physical circumstances that precede this moment, are perhaps a necessary condition, the act required to imprint the seal of life on the work of generation: like an electrified body, the seminal molecules perhaps receive in this way properties that they did not previously possess.[22]

Roussel follows up this scientific language with a reference to the folk belief that extramarital sex produces a better quality child, one more intelligent and spirited. Lovers who come together solely out of passion, we are to understand, exhibit none of the "inertia of soul" said by Roussel to characterize the marriage bed. Roussel concludes that "the ideas of the vulgar are not always to be disdained" (261).

Not that Julie is to be imagined writhing in the throes of sensual pleasure. Saint-Preux insists time and again on the languorousness of her lovemaking— she faints, he burns. A virtuous European woman is "passively" orgasmic, a contradiction in terms unless we consider descriptions such as the following from Buffon, in which "moment of conception" should be understood as equivalent to "orgasm":

---

[22]   Pierre Roussel, *Système physique et moral de la femme* (Paris: Vincent, 1775), 258. Future references in the text.

Women feel a sort of thrill throughout their body at the moment of conception, according to Hippocrates, and this shudder is strong enough to make their teeth clack together, like in a fever. Galen explains this symptom as the contraction and squeezing of the womb, and adds that women have told him that they felt this sensation when they conceived; other authors describe it as a slight feeling of cold that runs through the body.[23]

While the fruit of Julie and Saint-Preux's union might have been a truly exceptional child, society again trumps nature in this novel, for a miscarriage brought on by her father's violence quickly dashes Julie's hopes of forcing a marriage with Saint-Preux. The scene in which Julie's father first hits her, causing her to fall violently, then comforts her on his knees, is one of the strangest in the book, and would seem to enact the return to the Law of the Father that this novel has so often been said to represent.[24] One can also propose more pedestrian reasons for the miscarriage: the fetus may have been insecurely "fastened," for example. Roussel declares that widows and unmarried girls are prone to miscarriages, "and the reason for this is not difficult to discern" (249). Anxiety causes the embryos to attach to the wrong location, from which they are easily dislodged. Simon Boy's list of the causes of miscarriage include a fall such as Julie experiences, but the extent of his list makes any full-term pregnancy, whatever the psychological state of the mother, appear quite unlikely: "falls, blows, frights, violent passions of the soul, such as anger, etc., conjugal activity, coughs, vomiting, excessive exercise, overly heavy burdens, etc."[25]

Transcending the Female Condition

While Julie contemplates other strategies to force a marriage with Saint-Preux, the novel reaches a crucial turning point: Mme d'Etange discovers Saint-Preux's letters and learns of her daughter's affair. Already weakened by illness, Julie's mother is overcome by this revelation and quickly succumbs. Out of fear of causing the death of her remaining parent, Julie agrees to marry Wolmar, a nobleman who had once saved her father's life. She writes to ask Saint-Preux to free her from her promise to remain ever faithful to him. As with the scene in the *cabinet*, this letter overcomes the retrospective passiveness of the epistolary form by having Julie enact her message as she writes. As the ellipses in her missive indicate, Julie is

---

[23]   George-Louis Leclerc, comte de Buffon, *Histoire naturelle, générale et particulière*, 36 vols (Paris: Imprimerie Royale, 1749–1788), II:511–12.

[24]   See Tony Tanner, "Julie and 'La Maison Paternelle': Another Look at Rousseau's *La Nouvelle Héloïse*," in *The Family in Political Thought*, ed. Jean Bethke Eshtain (Amherst: University of Massachusetts Press, 1982).

[25]   Simon Boy, *Abrégé sur les maladies des femmes grosses, et de celles qui sont accouchées ... et la manière de soigner et traiter les enfans, depuis la naissance jusques vers l'âge de puberté* (Paris: Croullebois, 1788), 38.

inscribing her physical condition into the letter. In addition to the pen said to fall from her hand as she instructs her lover to stay away, these ellipses signify illness and signal to the reader that Saint-Preux will surely disobey:

> The pen falls from my hand. I have been unwell for several days; the discussion [with my father] this morning agitated me prodigiously … my head and my stomach hurt … I feel faint … will Heaven have pity on my sufferings? … I can no longer hold on … I am forced to get into bed, and console myself with the hope of never rising again. Adieu, my only love. (328)

"A headache," "sick to her stomach": these and other symptoms, including a high fever, indicate that Julie is suffering through the onset of smallpox. Once again, we are to understand, psychological trauma has led to illness. As will be clear in the upcoming scene of the "inoculation of love," in which Saint-Preux kisses Julie's pox-covered hand and thus ensures his own severe bout with the disease, smallpox was attributed to contagion in eighteenth-century France, however distrustful some remained of inoculation. Rousseau's instructions for the print of this scene indeed specify that Saint-Preux "must not only have no fear of contamination by the poison, he must desire it."[26] But how has Julie herself contracted the disease?

Voltaire addresses this question by transposing carrier and infected victim, advising us to understand this episode as a veiled reference to Julie's infection with that greater pox, syphilis, a "bitter" essence that she would have absorbed from Saint-Preux.[27] This metaphorical reading was part of a greater scheme to discredit Rousseau's claims to virtue by associating his well-known urinary troubles with the symptoms of syphilis. Voltaire's interpretation of Julie's illness is not supported, needless to say, by the spirit of Rousseau's novel. In a letter written to Saint-Preux after her recovery (and after her marriage to Wolmar), Julie offers the following etiology:

> You know, my friend; my health, so robust in the face of fatigue and the assaults of the air, has no resistance to the tempests of the passions; the source of all the ills that afflict my body and soul is my too sensitive heart. Whether distress, suffered over time, corrupted my blood; or nature chose that moment to purify it of a deadly germ, I felt terribly unwell at the end of that discussion [with my father]. (351)

Rousseau's depiction of Julie's sickness may have been inspired by vitalist theory or may have been written to reflect a general eighteenth-century vision of this much researched menace, one that would have been easily recognized by his readers. In either case, his reference to "a deadly germ" present in Julie's body and the "moment" chosen by nature to purify her body is strikingly vitalist in

---

[26]   Rousseau, *Sujets d'estampes*, in *Oeuvres complètes*, II:765.
[27]   Voltaire, *Lettres sur* La Nouvelle Héloïse, 407. Voltaire makes further reference to Saint-Preux's syphilis in the article "Bourreau" of the *Dictionnaire Philosophique*.

content and tone. The need to combat smallpox by inoculation was something of a vitalist obsession, an interest inspired among other factors by the outbreak that killed around two thousand victims in Montpellier in 1744. Bordeu's description of how "the germ" of smallpox grows only when it finds a fertile bodily field was published several years after the *New Heloise*, but the passage is worth citing in this context given its close alignment with the self-diagnosis offered to the reader by Rousseau's heroine:

> This [smallpox] seed germinates in the living body and eventually achieves a perfect maturity, reproducing and multiplying there; it is a physical cause that must find in the body into which it falls a particular disposition enabling it to grow and multiply. Properly speaking, this disposition is the medical cause of smallpox [as] without it the germ of small pox has utterly no effect on the body.[28]

The unidentified author of the *Encyclopédie* article "Smallpox (Medicine)" notes that this disease can either be transmitted by contact with another sufferer, or develop autonomously from a "germ" contained within the patient's own body, a latent infection that may have been present since birth. A chance circumstance such as a change in the air may cause this germ to erupt—the *Encyclopédie* article notes that smallpox is particularly virulent in the spring—but we know from her own testimony that Julie's "robust" natural health protects her from such "assaults of the air." We are left to conclude that a different "chance circumstance" (*cause occasionnelle*) has set the scene for the eruption of her illness, and the *Encyclopédie* provides an explanation: "A fright that is felt all the more strongly in that it is difficult to express; one knows only too well by experience the effect of the passions on our bodies and our humors."[29] The eruption of Julie's disease is thus to be understood as psychogenic, as she herself indicates by her reference to the "storm" (*intempérie*) of her passions. The *Dictionnaire de l'Académie* of 1762 notes that *intempérie* "is used only of the air and of the humors of the human body"; we are thus to understand that a stormy passion, like an infectious miasma, can bring on the worst of diseases.

Julie's retrospective letter is significant for more than her self-diagnosis, for it is in this missive that she gives Saint-Preux an account of their love affair while declaring it definitively over. Although she had agreed to marry Wolmar in the discussion with her father that had brought on her fever, she had later, as she convalesced, promised Saint-Preux the rights to her love even after her marriage.

---

[28] As cited by Elizabeth A. Williams, *A Cultural History of Medical Vitalism in Enlightenment Montpellier* (Ashgate, UK and Burlington, VT: Ashgate, 2003), 222, from Théophile de Bordeu, *Recherches sur quelques points de l'histoire de la médecine, qui peuvent avoir rapport à l'arrêt de la Grand'Chambre au Parlement de Paris, concernant l'inoculation et qui paroissent favorables à la tolérance de cette opération* (Liège/Paris: Cailleau, 1764), 162.

[29] "Vérole, petite, (Médec.)" in *Encyclopédie, ou Dictionnaire raisonné des sciences, des arts et des métiers*, ed. Denis Diderot and Jean d'Alembert (Paris: Briasson [etc.], 1751–1765), XVII:81.

She now finds such an arrangement intolerable, for on hearing the marriage vows pronounced, she tells Saint-Preux: "I believed that I felt a sudden interior revolution. An unknown power seemed suddenly to correct the disorder of my affections and reestablish them according to the laws of duty and of nature" (354).

The terms in which this "transformation" is described are strikingly medical, and recall Julie's conjecture that smallpox may have declared itself in her because "nature chose that moment to purify [my body] of a deadly germ" (351). The physical germ may have been expelled, but there was still, we understand by her agreement to continue her affair with Saint-Preux after marrying another, a serious moral peril present in Julie. Her humoral system as a whole is still at risk, until this moment of "interior revolution," a term that recalls the transformation at puberty that makes an adult young woman of a previously unformed child. What has caused this astounding reordering of Julie's "affections" into a calm and accepting state—reminiscent of that experienced by Saint-Preux in the high Alps? Given the setting—a marriage ceremony, a church—we can only conclude that a supernatural force has intervened to establish such an unlikely moral equilibrium despite the false, "unnatural" social context of the marriage.

Guillemette Johnston has read this scene as a submission to the social contract, arguing that Julie's reference to the "solemn knot of marriage" is a "tacit engagement with the human race to respect this sacred union."[30] Johnston's convincing reading makes Julie's decision to remain faithful to Wolmar an instance of submission to the "general will" as much as to providential intervention, but in any case, we are also to understand that some quasi-mysterious force has allowed Julie to suppress her passion for Saint-Preux and begin married life reconciled to her society's dictates. Rousseau then draws a chaste veil over the early years of Julie's married life, which take place in the silent interlude between the two parts of this novel. Sex with Wolmar, the birth of her two children, all of these important physical events are passed over in silence, presumably in that they offer little to none of the passion and excitement of Julie's premarriage existence. Only Saint-Preux's reappearance occasions the long discourses on the hygienic life enjoyed by the Wolmar family at Clarens that characterize the second part of the work, at least up until the moment of Julie's accidental near drowning and subsequent death.

When the ex-lovers meet again six years after Julie's wedding—a meeting arranged by Wolmar—their smallpox scars are the only physical legacy of their love. Saint-Preux, who had last seen Julie when he deliberately contracted her disease, describes this meeting in letter IV.6, written to Milord Edouard. While he had worried over the changes the years might have wrought to Julie's beauty, Saint-Preux had been especially fearful that smallpox might have marred her face: "My imagination stubbornly rejected the idea of marks on this charming face, and as soon as I conjured one scarred by smallpox, it was no longer that of Julie" (419). He is shocked to discover her yet more beautiful: "I saw with a surprise both

---

[30]   Guillemette Johnston, "The Divided Self in *La Nouvelle Héloïse*," *Studies on Voltaire and the Eighteenth Century* 278 (1999): 281.

bitter and sweet that she was actually more beautiful and more brilliant than ever." She is rounder, as befits her status as mother of two children, but this roundness only adds to her "blinding whiteness." While all of her features have no doubt filled out, we should understand this increased roundness as well as this stunning whiteness to apply to her now maternal chest, for we learn from Saint-Preux that Julie's face has indeed been marked by smallpox, albeit lightly: "Smallpox left on her cheeks only some almost imperceptible traces" (421).

In his note to this passage, the editor Bernard Guyon changes this phrase to "imperceptible traces," stating that only Saint-Preux has been scarred.[31] An "imperceptible trace" is a contradiction in terms, of course, but the exact level of Julie's scarring is indeed difficult to determine. We are perhaps to understand that while her complexion has suffered somewhat in its fineness, there are no clearly visible pockmarks. While recovering from the disease, Julie had expressed to Claire the hope that severe scarring would make her repugnant to Wolmar: "If I am able to reconcile myself to living, it is because I hope not to have escaped death entirely. My attractive face, for which my heart has paid so dearly, is no more" (328). Claire counters this notion by remarking that her own bout with the disease had caused greater scarring: "You suffered a cruel attack, but your face was spared. What you take for scars are only red marks that will soon disappear. I was left far worse than you, and you see, nonetheless, that I am still not all that unattractive" (334).

In *Smallpox and the Literary Imagination*, David Shuttleton cites many fictional examples of his observation that "a disfigured bride or wife tested the limits of male fidelity," and notes that Samuel Richardson's Pamela is left unmarked by her bout with smallpox.[32] Rousseau was in real life, apparently, an exception to this fictional rule, for according to the *Confessions* he passionately sought the company of Mme d'Houdetot, in whom he saw his Julie come-to-life: "Mme la comtesse d'Houdetot was approaching thirty and not at all beautiful. Her face was marked by smallpox, her complexion was not fine."[33] Whatever the exact degree of the fictional Julie's scarring, her fiancé did not reject her, as she had hoped: "M. de Wolmar arrived and was not discouraged by the change in my face" (353).

Saint-Preux's case is not at all equivocal, for we are to understand that he was severely marked by his own self-imposed illness. When Julie writes to Claire to describe her own reaction to their first meeting after six years of absence, she declares herself simultaneously repulsed and fascinated by these pockmarks: "His complexion is unrecognizable; he is 'as black as a Moor,' and badly scarred by smallpox. My dear, I must tell you everything: these marks are hard for me to look upon, and I often catch myself gazing at them" (427–8). Claire responds that Saint-Preux could "wear no more dangerous makeup," a claim clearly justified by the origin of his scars.

---

[31]   Jean-Jacques Rousseau, *Oeuvres complètes*, II:1594, note.

[32]   David Shuttleton, *Smallpox and the Literary Imagination, 1660–1820* (Cambridge: Cambridge University Press, 2007), 123.

[33]   Rousseau, *Confessions*, 439.

But even without the sacrifice signified by these scars, Saint-Preux's marks would not necessarily take away from his attractiveness, for Shuttleton observes that in Frances Brooke's *The History of Emily Montagu* (1769) the heroine falls for a man whose scars are said to give him a sensible, manly, even gentlemanly look: "Unlike the prevalent narrative of the scarred woman condemned to social death, a degree of facial scarring on a man could be represented as conferring character, sustaining if not increasing his social stature."[34]

Claire interprets the relative scarring experienced by the two lovers as any good reader should, metaphorically, albeit with a theological twist. She interprets the variation in the ex-lovers' facial scarring as a test set by God to try their respective virtues. Saint-Preux's many scars are so many enduring signifiers of his continuing, inextinguishable love for Julie, and therefore Julie as well easily recognizes them as a temptation to adultery. Should her own face have been heavily scarred however, this disfiguration would have lessened her fatal attractiveness to Saint-Preux. Despite his continuing adoration for her, he himself recognizes this possibility. Claire reaffirms that Julie has no or very little scarring years after her illness: "No doubt Heaven wished that he be marked by this illness in order to test your virtue, and that you be unmarked, in order to test his" (434).

Divinely orchestrated temptation aside, there is another possible interpretation for this striking difference. Saint-Preux deliberately inoculated himself with smallpox as an expression of his love, a love he never attempted to repress. Julie's smallpox erupted from within as the result of severe shock coupled with acute guilt. Claire describes Julie just before her outbreak as a woman whose internal flow of humors is so sluggish as to affect her mental functioning, painting a terrifying portrait of this calm-before-the-storm: "Her heart seems oppressed by affliction, and this excess of feeling that attacks her gives her an air of stupidity more frightening than sharp cries" (307). Claire's description fits Daignan's account of the physical symptoms that accompany a "great passion," as he refers to any strong emotional blow: "A universal upheaval, followed by frightening symptoms that announce the sufferings of nature. The face grows pale, the heart beats fast, the members tremble; the extremities stiffen, the entire body is covered with sweat and becomes sticky, and movement ceases; the sufferer returns to life in the midst of convulsions" (287).

While this oppression brought on by guilt will manifest itself as smallpox pustules after Julie's mother dies, the "almost imperceptible" level of scarring that results testifies that our heroine's sense of culpability, however strongly felt, was ultimately unfounded. My reading of Julie's scars is backed up by Rousseau-the-editor, who in a footnote places blame for the affair above all on Julie's mother. In her husband's absence, Mme d'Etange had engaged a young man as her daughter's tutor, and the inevitable occurred; she therefore bears the blame: "The two lovers are to be pitied; only the mother is inexcusable" (85). Mme d'Etange's sudden death is to be understood, in spite of Julie's feelings of shame and responsibility,

---

[34] Shuttleton, *Smallpox*, 158.

as brought on less by shock at what her daughter has done than by guilt at what she herself has allowed to happen, in combination with an innately weak constitution.

Julie's scars would similarly be "almost imperceptible" if we view them as so many signs of her continuing love for Saint-Preux, so violently repressed during the "interior revolution" that took place on her wedding day. Aware of the potential eruption of such powerful internal forces, Julie's husband, the wise, materialist Wolmar, treats the reunion of the two lovers as something of an exercise in disease control. As Julie relates the tale to Claire in letter IV.13, Wolmar begins by telling the two ex-lovers his life story. He then informs them that he has known of their affair since before his marriage to Julie and has always admired them for the singular nature of their love. They may have been led by a "false enthusiasm," but such passions only affect "beautiful souls." Wolmar continues by explaining that he has always understood that "there were connections between you that were not to be broken; that your mutual attachment was formed by so many admirable things, that it was rather to be regulated than destroyed ... I knew that great struggles only irritate great passions" (495). He has actively worked to reunite Julie and Saint-Preux so that they will see each other as the friends they have now become. Having told his story, he leads them to the famous *bosquet* and has them kiss again, to quite different effect. Julie writes: "This kiss was nothing like the one that had made this grove so redoubtable. I sadly congratulated myself, and I knew that my heart was more changed than I had dared to believe until that moment" (496).

The fire of their youthful passion has gone the way of their pristine visages and Julie's nubile breasts; gone are the half-faints, and the exclamations that Julie's kisses are "too bitter, too penetrating; they pierce, they burn" (65). Having conceived the project of making Saint-Preux his children's tutor, Wolmar needs a complete cure and thus takes a trip during which the ex-lovers, left together at Clarens with no husband to oversee their kisses, will be put to a lengthier, more difficult test. The experiment works, for after a visit to the "rocks of Meillerie," the scene of one of his most passionate attacks of love for Julie, Saint-Preux realizes what Wolmar already knows: the woman he loves is the young Julie of his dreams, who no longer exists. Saint-Preux declares in letter VI.7 that his "cure" is now complete: "When this redoubtable Julie pursues me, I take refuge near Madame de Wolmar and I am tranquil" (677).

The most unlikely aspect of Saint-Preux's behavior is that he chooses to remain faithful to this oneiric Julie. His sexual fidelity must be placed however in the context of the heightened physical suffering Saint-Preux experienced during their love affair. In a metaphorization of his smallpox scars, Saint-Preux declares that the marks left by these "wounds of love" form a tight seal: "The wound is healed, but the mark remains, and this mark is the respected seal that preserves the heart from another attack. Inconstancy and love are incompatible" (675). The bitter fires of his passion have "reduced" him to a pure essence, insuring an unnatural type of fidelity quite different from that resulting from Julie's process of purification, cited above: "No, no, the fires with which I burned purified me; I am no longer in any way an ordinary man" (678). He thus resists Julie's efforts to arrange another relationship for him: "Do not seek to awaken me from the numbness into which I have fallen; for fear that along with the feeling of my own existence, I also regain the old sufferings, and that this violent state then reopens all my wounds" (681).

What of Julie, whose "wounds of love" have left few, if any, visible marks? She declares herself perfectly happy; she has achieved everything she needs, and is ready for death: "O death, come when you will! I no longer fear you" (689). Somewhat unnecessarily, the "editor" intervenes to point out the contradiction inherent in such a statement, although Rousseau's note also allows him to qualify this letter as Julie's "swan song," and thus to hint that her death is indeed imminent (694). Our heroine has one foot out of this world already, for as she reveals to Saint-Preux, the "perfect" earthly happiness she has obtained is less-than-satisfying in the spiritual realm. She frequently seeks refuge from this "perfection" in her *cabinet*, in order to "refill" her empty soul: "By rising to the source of feeling and being, [my soul] loses its dryness and languor: it is reborn, reanimated" (694). She is using devotion as a medicine, carefully calibrated: "Too strong a dose puts you to sleep, makes you mad, or kills you; I hope not to go that far" (697). Julie had predicted this scenario, for soon after they first made love, she wrote to tell Saint-Preux:

> I see, my friend, by the stamp of our souls and our common tastes, that love will be the great affair of our lives. When once it has left the profound impressions that we have received, it must extinguish or absorb all the other passions; the slightest cooling would be for us the languor of death; an invincible distaste, an eternal ennui, would succeed the end of our love, and we would not live long after ceasing to love. (109)

That Julie's "antidote" is acting against the particular disease of "love," made chronic, although latent, by early exposure, becomes clear only when she is on her deathbed. There is a physical explanation given for her death: she becomes ill after jumping into the water to save her young son, Marcellin, who had slipped off the dike on which they were strolling. That physiologists such as Roussel will later cite a woman's ability to "throw herself into the waves" after her drowning child as proof that they rely more on instinct than reason, and thus make better, more self-sacrificing caregivers, may be a sign of the novel's popularity, but Julie attributes her untimely end to the intervention of a providential hand. In her last, famous letter to Saint-Preux (VI.12), she reveals that her love for him has resurfaced in all its intensity now that she knows herself to be dying. The passion she believed to have been quite thoroughly purged had remained within her, and might well have resurfaced in all its virulent intensity under the influence of the circumstance (*cause occasionnelle*) of Saint-Preux's long-term installation at Clarens as tutor to her children. But now she is dying and thus, paradoxically, out of danger: "I fooled myself for a long time. This illusion was salutary; it disappeared only when I no longer needed it … My friend, I admit this feeling with no shame; it remained in me involuntarily, and it has in no way affected my innocence" (740–41).

There are significant similarities between the section of the novel that details Julie's bout with smallpox and that describing her final illness. In a letter from

Wolmar to Saint-Preux (VI.11) in which Julie's death is described at length, we are told that during the fevered night that convinces her doctor she will indeed soon die, she calls out not only for Marcellin, but also for "another name, once so often repeated on a similar occasion" (706). The theme of the disfigured face returns as well in a letter from Julie to Saint-Preux: "When you see this letter, the worm will be gnawing the face of your lover, and her heart, where you will be no longer" (743). This sentence, read in isolation, might seem horrifically morbid, for even if the ravaged face of Julie's decaying corpse is read as signifying the intensity of her repressed passion for Saint-Preux, he will be quite thoroughly absent, she tells him, from her decaying heart. What transforms this statement is our knowledge that "heart" is to be understood here as the now lifeless organ. In the last pages of this novel, Rousseau emphasizes the one rather unorthodox belief of this otherwise conformist Christian woman: Julie does not accept the resurrection of the body (letter VI.11). As she had written to Saint-Preux, her love for him had been like a hidden germ of illness, "concentrated in her heart"; she is now happily convinced that she will soon leave her physical body behind for good when she dies, and enter unblemished into God's fold. In this setting, her love for Saint-Preux will be purified of its sinful possibilities, and thus able to coexist peacefully with her love for her husband and her duty to her father. Her worm-eaten face, like her empty heart, will signify nothing blameworthy once her soul leaves her body.

Unfortunately, those simpler souls who surround Julie at Clarens and worship her as a near saint do not share her transcendental philosophy. A rumor that she has undergone a Christ-like physical resurrection causes a near riot (her father's superstitious servant imagines that he sees Julie's corpse open its eyes and nod to him). Wolmar is afraid to remove his wife's body from her bed, and the gruesome result is that her corpse begins to decompose in full view of her loved ones. Wolmar describes this process in his letter to Saint-Preux: "Her flesh was beginning to decay, and although her face retained her sweet features, one saw in it already some signs of alteration." Claire finally brings an end to the hysteria by placing a veil over Julie's face and declaiming: "Cursed be the unworthy hand that ever lifts this veil! Cursed be the impious eye that ever looks upon this disfigured face!" (737).

In other words, we as readers are again instructed, by means of what might otherwise seem merely an unfortunate, grisly digression, to look elsewhere for the purely spiritual version of Julie we have seen evolving throughout this novel. Death is the final liberation for her, as her soul will no longer be bound to her body. As she lies on her deathbed, Julie declares herself already liberated from the duality that had ruled her life: "My body still lives, but my moral life is over. I am at the end of my career and already judged on my past. To suffer and die is all that remains for me; that is the business of nature" (716). The dichotomy between nature and culture, so important to Rousseau's social and moral philosophy, is perhaps nowhere in his writings so strikingly delineated as in Julie's death scene. With her physical being caught in the throes of its agonal struggle, she feels herself freed not only from the desires of her body but also from the greater evil of civilized social intercourse, and thus from the possibility of sin.

Julie's triumphant apotheosis would have no meaning, and would have been quite unsatisfactory to eighteenth-century readers, had she not first worked her way through the Valley of the Shadow. Her life story, in other words, is an exemplary response to the question posed and answered by her fellow youthful sinner, the Savoyard vicar: "Why is my soul subjected to my senses and chained to this body that dominates and irritates it?" The vicar explains that without the temptations of the flesh, humans would be mere angels, and would lack both the merit of a struggle overcome, and the greater glory and happiness of tested virtue.[35] As readers of *The New Heloise*, we are to conclude with the vicar that only through the limitations of temporary symbiosis with a body can the immortal soul experience the unique spiritual exercise otherwise known as life.[36] No *Valaisanne*, that is, could equal Julie's hard-won virtue.

It is this all-too-human capacity to triumph through suffering that Wolmar, the atheist, most admires in his wife, and this admiration explains his tolerance for Saint-Preux's presence in his home (a plot detail that was also, needless to say, irresistible fodder for Voltaire's mockery). Wolmar reveals that he himself had experienced passion only once in his life when, overcome by love and jealousy, he had agreed to separate Julie from her lover by marrying her. While the result was ultimately positive, his action holds no value in his eyes in that he had not demonstrated the courage necessary to resist her: "Only fiery souls are capable of combating and vanquishing. All great efforts, all sublime actions, are their work" (493). The act of throwing herself in the water to save her child at the cost of her own life was unimpressive, for her husband, compared to how Julie faced her death: "Other mothers might leap in to save their children. Accident, fever, death, all are a part of nature: such is the common fate of mortals; but the use of her last moments, her speeches, her feelings, her soul, all of that belongs to Julie alone" (704).

That Julie was the subject of such rapturous and continuous admiration from her husband Wolmar, her best friend Claire, and her ex-lover Saint-Preux may go a long way toward explaining her popularity with eighteenth-century women readers. She is both an appealingly transcendent character and, by virtue of her premarital affair with Saint-Preux, a heroine on a human scale. Her redemption, sanctioned, significantly, by her husband, would certainly have made her more palatable to women readers as well. To conclude this chapter, I consider the ways in which Julie differs from the heroines of well-known novels by eighteenth-women that consider similar themes of a young woman caught in a loveless marriage and forced to adapt to an "unnatural" situation. The first point to be made is that Julie's loss of physical virtue is a plot device never included in the works of the great French women novelists of this period. Nor are their heroines tied to their bodies

---

35   Rousseau, *Emile*, 603.

36   For an overview of opinions on the novel's final pages, considered tragic and pessimistic by many commentators, see Anne Srabian de Fabry, "Quelques observations sur le dénouement de *La Nouvelle Héloïse*," in *Etudes autour de* La Nouvelle Héloïse (Québec: Editions Naaman de Sherbrooke, 1977), 19–29.

in the manner in which Julie is described as a product of her environment, down to the size of her breasts.

Women-authored novels possess their own version of the ideal eighteenth-century French woman, described in a manner quite incongruent with that of male authors. The heroines of novels by women writers tend to exhibit both the high sensibility and the instinctual virtue manifested by Julie, but they are to be viewed as unique and exceptional individuals, not as a miraculous "norm" of femininity. And while Julie's reasoned observations about her place in the world and the meaning of love and virtue are admirably developed, Rousseau never cites her capacity to reason objectively about the world as an integral part of her ideal status as a woman. It seems more of an outgrowth of her virtue than a characteristic feature. In the work of women writers the contention that the mind has no sex, but that the female sex is nevertheless far more instinctively virtuous than the other, is the implied but rarely stated basis for comparing male and female characters.

Riccoboni is the most useful example in this context for many reasons, including the popularity of her eight novels. She was born Marie-Jeanne de Heurles de Laboras in 1713. Her early life was marked by tragedy, for her father abandoned Marie-Jeanne and her mother in Paris after a conviction for bigamy required him to return to a first wife and family. As an illegitimate young girl, she was placed in a convent school and destined for the cloister. She rebelled against this fate and in 1734 married the actor Antoine-François Riccoboni. After acting for a time, she left the stage to write, and her novels were successful from the start. She began to frequent some of the most prestigious intellectual salons of the time, including that of d'Holbach, where she met Denis Diderot, among others. Her best-known works are *Letters of Mistress Fanny Butlerd* (1757), *The Story of M. le Marquis de Cressy* (1758), *Letters of Milady Juliette Catesby* (1759), and *The Story of Ernestine* (1765), all more or less contemporary to Rousseau's *Julie or the New Heloise* (1761).

Riccoboni's novels have been characterized as feminist in great part for her depiction of sensitive, intelligent women who suffer at the hands of brutish or merely insensitive men, but critics have also recently pointed to the strong philosophical element in her works as an attempt by a woman writer to pick apart the meaning of gender difference in the Enlightenment.[37] Among these critics is Heidi Bostic, who has argued for the reasoned nature of the solutions Riccoboni's female characters find for the problems created by their living in "a society organized to their disadvantage."[38] Among these "reasoned solutions" is the

---

[37] On the issue of Riccoboni's feminism, see Colette Cazenobe, "Le Féminisme paradoxal de Madame Riccoboni," *Revue d'histoire littéraire de la France* 88 (1988): 23–45; Andrée Demay, *Marie-Jeanne Riccoboni ou de la pensée féministe chez une romancière du XVIIIᵉ siècle* (Paris: Pensée Universelle, 1977); and Felicia Sturzer, "Epistolary and Feminist Discourse: Julie de Lespinasse and madame Riccoboni," *Studies on Voltaire and the Eighteenth Century* 304 (1992): 739–42.

[38] Heidi Bostic, *The Fiction of Enlightenment: Women of Reason in the French Eighteenth Century* (Newark: University of Delaware Press, 2010), 106.

suicide of the wife of the title character of *The Story of M. le Marquis de Cressy*. Madame la Marquise has every reason to be unhappy with her husband, for she has discovered that he married her only for her money, that he had attempted to rape a young woman before their marriage, and that he has been having an affair with an orphaned adolescent they have taken into their home. She kills herself through the intermediary of this eminently guilty spouse, asking him to hand her a cup of tea into which she has put poison.

Bostic argues that this carefully planned death is to be viewed as based on the Socratic model of philosophically accepting one's fate, rather than as the desperate act of a hysterical woman. Suicide was a highly charged subject for Riccoboni's Christian readers, of course, and Bostic points out that at least one other woman writer found the suicide of the Marquise to be morally revolting. Another reviewer declared the act lacking in verisimilitude for a woman painted as highly virtuous throughout the novel. Such a violent end is simply not womanly, by eighteenth-century standards, but the point of the novel, as Bostic argues, is precisely the virile courage with which this virtuous woman faces her death and the symbolic responsibility she so clearly places on her husband by having him unwittingly hand her the poisoned tea.[39]

I would add that the Marquise acts according to another model as well: that of the medical theories of her era. After learning of her ward's betrayal with her husband, the Marquise withdraws to the country and takes eight days to reach a decision. She diagnoses her condition as fatal, given that she feels her health rapidly deteriorating day by day. She knows her time on earth to be short and decides to cut it even shorter, making her death ultimately more euthanasia than suicide. Her references to the tea she will drink are particularly striking. When her ward Mlle de Berneil observes her putting a "white powder" into her cup, the Marquise tells the young woman who has betrayed her that the substance is a *calmant* "that will help me to rest." She then places it on the table so that the tea will be properly infused with these "calming" properties.

When her husband arrives, the Marquise asks Berneil to stay and her husband to fill her cup completely. As he hands it to her, she declares: "I am charmed, monsieur, to take this salutary remedy from you."[40] After allowing the poison to work, she hands each witness to her death an envelope and begins a prepared speech. When her husband realizes what is happening, she counsels him to remain calm, adding that she is happy to have taken from his "once cherished hand" a no-fail cure (*un spécifique sûr*) for her "unbearable suffering" (298). She refuses medical treatment, declaring that it is too late. Her husband's reaction is satisfyingly dramatic and repentant. He takes his wife in his arms and kisses her—in the process revealing the *spécifique* that might have saved her, had it been administered early enough: "His caresses, his passionate expressions, brought

---

39   Bostic, *The Fiction of Enlightenment*, 124.

40   Marie-Jeanne Riccoboni, *Histoire du marquis de Cressy*, *Oeuvres* (Paris, Brissot-Thivars, 1826), I:296. Future references in the text.

madame de Cressy back to life; a lively color chased away her pallor; her sweet and charming traits regained all their splendor; joy was painted on her face" (300). He has administered this cure (learned his lesson) too late of course, leading to an equally satisfying dénouement. Berneil withdraws to a convent and the Marquis, having nearly died from despair, may go on to a life of wealth and honor but is said to be simultaneously made miserable by crushing guilt and unhappiness (301).

The "transformation" Julie undergoes during her Church wedding in order to become a faithful wife to a husband who adores her (however coldly rational he may be) seems quite thoroughly passive in comparison to the marquise de Cressy's "solution" to her problems. When faced with impossible situations, Julie collapses in a psychogenic illness, such as the wretched state that caused her friend Claire to recall Saint-Preux and create the context for an inevitable physical consummation of their affair. Her smallpox is of course the most dramatic example of how her body literally shuts down in the face of stressful decisions, and her hope that the resulting scars will chase off her suitor Wolmar reveals a reliance on passive resistance that is characteristic of Julie's virtue. Rousseau grants her a wise husband whose knowledge of hygiene allows her a long, relatively calm existence at Clarens, during which the passion she felt for her lover, already repressed by divine intervention, is allowed to remain quite thoroughly latent until her imminent death permits it to resurface with no threat to her virtue. The marquise de Cressy's situation is, needless to say, far more dire, and her reaction once she finally grasps the full horror of her husband's behavior is not only forceful and rational, as Bostic has argued, but also seconded by the use of medical terminology designed to place her "suicide" in the realm of self-diagnosis and necessary self-medication.

Another example of a female character from a novel by an eighteenth-century woman writer reinforces the differences between Julie's fate and that of her fictional sisters. The *Letters of Mistress Henley Published by Her Friend* by the Swiss writer Isabelle de Charrière ends with the heroine warning the woman friend to whom she has been writing that "in a year, or two, you will learn, I hope, that I am reasonable and contented, or that I am no more."[41] Mistress Henley's use of *raisonnable* in this final paragraph of the novel's last letter would seem to indicate that the married heroine views herself as having until this point behaved like a child in that she lacked "reason," a deficit, one might conclude, that is the cause of both her unhappiness and her (possibly) imminent death, should she not rectify it. But the novel makes it quite clear that Mistress Henley has an eminently reasonable understanding of her situation and that if she were to die it would be from the unbearable prospect of living with an overly "reasonable" man, not any lack of intelligence or intellectual ability on her own part. To be become "reasonable" in the sense she is using it would mean to deny her innate *sensibilité*, a characteristic by no means negative for the period, of course.

---

[41]   Isabelle de Charrière, *Lettres de Mistriss Henley publiées par son amie* (New York: Modern Language Association, 1993), 45.

Mister Henley's cold moderation in all things, we learn through the course of the novel, has made it impossible for him to have the sentimental relationship with his wife that she so desperately craves. Mistress Henley thus faces a situation at least as impossible as Julie's, for she must either excise all feeling from her heart in order to be a better match for her husband, or die of the sheer despair of living with and for a man who has no understanding whatsoever of her rich inner life and no intention of meeting her halfway. She stresses that she will not kill herself, but adds that "sadness" can kill. The novel's title—letters from Mistress Henley published by her friend—is meant to indicate to the reader that Mistress Henley did not achieve her goal of excising all feeling from her heart and is therefore no more. That the last letter of this monophonic epistolary work is indeed the "last letter" ever received by the *amie* is made clear by our holding the book in our hands.

These two women-authored deaths—only one clearly a suicide, but both ascribable to a serious character flaw on the part of a husband that leads to physical collapse and death on the part of a wife—are in sharp contrast to Julie's pseudo-suicide. Julie may "own" her death after she is taken from the river, for she certainly does not fight it, but the accident that nearly drowns her is framed by a motherly virtue so strong that it overcomes any religious doubts as to the voluntary nature of her death. The most dramatic consequence of her knowledge that she is dying is that she is able to allow her feelings for Saint Preux, "mystically" repressed during her wedding ceremony, to surface. In comparison to Cressy and Henley, Julie's intellect plays no role in the solution to her problems. It is her instinctual perfection, mirrored in her status as the perfect physiological specimen of femaleness, that makes her a superior woman and grants her the divine transformation necessary to reconcile her to a life without love.

Ultimately Julie transcends, rather than facing and dealing rationally with, the problems associated with marriage that were so realistically depicted by Rousseau, Riccoboni, and Charrière, and deadly in the novels of all three of these authors as well. Only Julie, however, and despite her transcendent qualities, is cut from the same cloth as the materialist descriptions of the feminine ideal in the era's hygiene treatises. Riccoboni and Charrière's heroines are not of course to be considered "intellectuals" in the full sense of that term, for they are like Julie characterized above all by a great degree of sensibility, an unlimited capacity to love, and an innate sense of virtue. What distinguishes them from Julie is that they must solve their own societally induced emotional problems rather than being whisked away to Clarens and the protection of a loving husband. Forced against the wall, these ideal feminine specimens manage to transcend their situations in an enviably rational manner and quite on their own. That a woman characterized exclusively by cold reason could only ever be a monster will be clear in the following chapter, in which the infamous marquise de Merteuil is analyzed from the point of view of her era's physiological theories and her own (mistaken, I argue) assumptions about how nature's desires continue to be felt in the confused hearts and minds of civilized men and women.

Chapter 4
The Marquise de Merteuil,
or Sexuality in the State of Nature

In vain do the prideful wish to pity natural woman her fate; she possesses liberty,
strength, health, beauty, and love. What more does she need to be happy?
          —Choderlos de Laclos, "On Women and Their Education"

Dangerous Liaisons (1782), Choderlos de Laclos's only novel, is considered by
most critics to be the greatest epistolary novel produced during the century most
devoted to this genre. I would add to this accolade that *Dangerous Liaisons* ranks
as the most biting fictional commentary on the level of degradation present in late
eighteenth-century French culture. This cultural decadence is of course personified
in the novel by a woman, Mme de Merteuil. The *divine marquise* is a complex,
multifaceted character, whose fictional motives are often quite difficult if not
impossible for a reader to discern. Without the help of an omniscient narrator, the
reader of this epistolary tour-de-force knows only that Merteuil takes extraordinary
care in writing her letters and that her central focus in composing any missive is
to manipulate its recipient.

As readers we can, however, make some observations as to how Merteuil
accomplishes these machinations, and more importantly, we can attempt to
outline the philosophy behind her actions. As a libertine, Merteuil believes that
men and women are driven above all by sexual desire, but that lesser human
beings are unable to admit this basic truth even to themselves. For Merteuil, this
disconnection between desire and morality—between the physical and moral—is
a boon, for it makes those around her quite easy to manipulate. The most deluded
of these individuals, she tells her ex-lover and confidante the vicomte de Valmont,
are those women who hide behind the lie of love, "whose exalted imaginations
make them believe that nature placed their sensations in their heads; and who,
having never reflected on the matter, always confuse love for their lover."[1] But
while these women have foolishly accepted what they have been taught from a
young age—to value the hypocritical veneer of modesty promoted by their society
as the highest element of their natures—Merteuil, we are to understand, knows
better and operates under no such limitations.

In this chapter, I argue that while *Dangerous Liaisons* is certainly a condemnation
of the decadence of eighteenth-century French culture, this novel is at the same
time an homage to the resilience of nature's beneficent influence. By the end of the
novel we are to realize that despite her apparent triumphs, Merteuil is quite simply

---

[1]   Choderlos de Laclos, *Liaisons dangereuses*, in *Oeuvres complètes* (Paris: Gallimard,
1979), 170. Future references in the text.

wrong in her assumptions about the human condition. The ultimate proof of her faulty vision is that however successful she may be at using others as her unwitting pawns, she botches the endgame. The cause of her downfall and disfigurement as recounted in the last letters of the novel is her severe underestimation of the role that love plays in the civilized state. Laclos directly addresses the role of love in human sexuality in his 1783 essay "On Women and Their Education," in which he presents this emotion as an essential part of the sex act in the "state of nature." In a lengthy prolegomenon to his diagnosis of the crisis faced by contemporary French women, Laclos presents monogamy and fidelity as quite thoroughly absent from "natural" relations between men and women, but insists that the (fleeting) experience of love is part of "natural" sexual behavior. He makes this argument as he traces the coming-to-puberty of a "natural" young girl who develops into a woman said to enjoy all the happiness granted by the "liberty, strength, health, beauty, and love" cited in the epigraph to this chapter, with the last item in this list the most important, for my purposes.[2]

Reading Laclos's essay in tandem with his novel, I argue that Merteuil's emotionally stunted view of human relationships—her valuation of power over not only love but sexual satisfaction as well—is to be understood as linked to her status as a physiologically and thus morally perverse variation on the female human being. Merteuil's association with decadence in this novel is, in other words, far more than a mere indictment of the aristocracy or of libertinage as a general philosophy. We are to see her as embodying the negative, distorting effects of the (too) high degree of civilization her social status confers upon her. Merteuil's physico-moral perversity is not however merely the result of her exposure to the decadent social practices of eighteenth-century Paris, as one might expect. We know that Merteuil's physiology is marked by an innate (possibly inherited) deformation rather than sabotaged at puberty because we are privy to the details of her passage through this "revolution," given in the famous autobiographical letter II.81. I argue that this letter is intended to alert the reader to the physiological irregularities that are responsible for both Merteuil's exceptional intellect and her mistaken views on the human condition. There is something missing in Merteuil, or perhaps something extra, and this element makes her a "monster" in the etymological sense of a "prodigy," something extraordinary that also functions as a warning.[3]

---

[2]   Choderlos de Laclos, "Des Femmes et de leur éducation," in *Oeuvres complètes*, 404. Future references in the text. Laclos wrote three essays on women, of which "Des Femmes" is the second. The first was a response (neither completed nor submitted) to a question on women's education posed by the Académie de Châlons-sur-Marne (1783). A third essay, probably written between 1795–1802, is said to have been composed at the request of la comtesse de Gurson and deals with the proper reading material for young girls.

[3]   Teratology was a subject of much fascination for eighteenth-century biologists, with a disturbance in the mother's psychological state most often given as the cause of congenital deformation. See Sander Gilman, *Sexuality: An Illustrated History* (New York: Wiley and Sons, 1989), 161–93. The use of monstrous births to further political ends is explored in *Monstrous Bodies/Political Monstrosities in Early Modern Europe* (2004).

I am hardly the first to view Merteuil as a "monster," but the monstrosity that I detect is of a physical nature, a flaw hidden by her beautiful exterior (we are never given a portrait in words of Merteuil, but her attractiveness is nevertheless made evident).[4] In adding a reading of Merteuil's physiology to the debate on her character, I present the connection between her physical and moral monstrousness as the vitalists configured all such associations: both intimate and causal. She is an exception to the vitalist rule however and all the more dangerous in that there are no outward manifestations of Merteuil's monstrosity until the novel's final letters. There are no exterior signs pointing to her inner corruption, and this absence allows the Marquise to function both as a bizarre and dangerous physiological phenomenon—an example of the mind–body link gone terribly wrong—and as a trope for the dangers of the overly civilized state. Merteuil personifies the glittering lifestyle of her era and her social class until her exposure as a moral monster coincides with her transformation into a physical monster at the end of the novel. She is the virus coursing, unseen, in the blood of her society—a medical analogy anachronistic only on the level of terminology, for at the novel's end, Merteuil's seemingly healthy body will be shown to have harbored (à la Julie), perhaps from birth, the latent germ of a disease that blossoms only when her moral perfidy is made public: the dreaded, disfiguring smallpox.

Puberty and the Female Monster

Londa Schiebinger notes that much of the argument concerning female physiology and sexual commensurability during the late eighteenth century was part of a growing ideological push to rein in the privileges of aristocratic women.[5] Given that both Merteuil and Valmont are manifestly members of the *noblesse d'épée*, or the most ancient of noble families, they represent a class in grave disrepute, with Merteuil's sex marking her as the more dangerous of the pair.[6] Their libertinism is in many ways an outgrowth of their social class and as such a symptom of what ails their society. Critics have viewed Merteuil and Valmont as personifying

---

    [4] Merteuil's monstrosity has also been denied, notably by Suellen Diaconoff who argues that the ambiguity of Merteuil's character makes her all the more intensely human and "proves that Laclos was not aiming to present her as the symbol of any single value, such as intelligence or satanic evil, as certain critics maintain" (*Eros and Power in Les Liaisons dangereuses: A Study in Evil* [Geneva: Droz, 1979], 34).

    [5] Londa Schiebinger, *The Mind Has No Sex? Women in the Origins of Modern Science* (Cambridge, MA: Harvard University Press, 1989), 217.

    [6] It is not possible to determine exactly when the reader is to believe the letters that make up this novel were written; we are told in the "editor's" preface that they could not possible have been composed by contemporaries, for in "our" day, "we" would never see a young, wealthy girl retreat to a convent nor a "young and pretty" *Présidente* die of a broken heart (4).

both the acme and the ultimate failure of the libertine project, with Ernest Sturm, for example, placing the duo at the logical (dead) end of libertinism. For Sturm, this pair illustrates "the insufficiencies of a hedonism that triumphed during the Regency and that progressively degenerated into a sort of ferocious autolatry and misanthropy."[7] Jean Goldzink similarly qualifies the search for sexual pleasure by Laclos's libertines as devoid of the emphasis on moderation one finds in the earlier writings of authors such as Crébillon *fils*.[8]

Merteuil's libertinism is central to her characterization and to my analysis, but I differ from previous commentators in reversing cause and effect. Rather than viewing her "monstrousness" as having its source in a philosophy she willingly and rationally adopts, I argue that her libertinism is rather a symptom of how very much the Marquise deviates from the gendered norm of the "new woman." In great part, and despite the obvious appeal of her extraordinary character to many readers, Merteuil's expertise in dominating all the "lesser" beings who surround her is to be understood as the result of a physical aberration with profound consequences for her existence as a sexed being, in keeping with the physiology of puberty and female sexuality that reigned during the late eighteenth century.

Merteuil's conviction that she is the intellectual superior of any man makes her the perfect foil for the "new woman" of the two-sex model, as portrayed by Daignan, Roussel, and so many others. The Marquise is the opposite extreme from that highly reactive, innately coquettish creature, "delightfully" soft and round due to her swollen connecting tissue, slightly befuddled by reason of her equally plethoric brain. But while Merteuil's cold intelligence makes her a glorious exception to the limits placed on the female mind in such works, it also means that she ultimately cannot truly compete with her main female rival, the Présidente de Tourvel, for the affections of the vicomte de Valmont, for he is irresistibly drawn to Tourvel against his better (libertine) judgment. Tourvel is a Julie placed in the most decadent of all settings, Parisian haute society, making her all the more impossible according to the physiological theories of her day, and all the more ideal for that contradiction. Faced with this specimen of matchless femininity, all Merteuil can do is to cause Valmont to kill off her rival, inadvertently and thus all the more painfully for him, even though the result of this murder-by-proxy will be her own expulsion from society.

Taken together, Merteuil and Tourvel represent two extreme, dueling images of womanhood in this work: the stereotypical French aristocrat who has lost her femininity and seeks power above all other things and the Julie-like heroine who miraculously retains her natural female characteristics in spite of her depraved surroundings. While I will consider the Merteuil–Tourvel dynamic in the second part of this chapter, in this first part I concentrate on another female character who belongs quite squarely in the middle of this dialectic of extremes:

---

[7]   Ernest Sturm, *Crébillon fils ou la science du désir* (Paris: A. G. Nizet, 1995), 12.

[8]   Jean Goldzink, *Le Vice en bas de soie ou le roman du libertinage* (Paris: José Corti, 2001), 115–17.

Cécile Volanges, a young woman fresh from the convent who is clearly neither highly intelligent nor especially virtuous. Cécile is designed to play the role of the normal, fully blossomed, limited, weak-brained, postpubescent-yet-predefloration young woman of the hygiene treatises. As such, she is the weaker, civilized counterpart to the young girl in the state of nature who stars in "On Women and Their Education," written a year after the publication of *Dangerous Liaisons*.

That the young and innocent Cécile will be highly significant to the unfolding of the novel's plot is clear from the beginning, for Laclos assigns her the work's opening letter, written to a friend left behind under the protection of the nuns. We learn from this juvenile missive with its series of exclamations and unsophisticated surmises that Cécile is the very cliché of the young girl who has been given over to the care of unworldly souls. She is naive, grossly undereducated, and quite thoroughly ignorant of the mores of Parisian high society, that treacherous milieu into which she has just been thrown. Her fate is indeed sealed in the novel's second letter, from Merteuil to Valmont, in which we learn that the Marquise plans to use Cécile to take revenge on a certain Gercourt, Merteuil's ex-lover and Cécile's fiancé. Gercourt has committed the unpardonable sin of leaving Merteuil of his own volition, rather than being manipulated into believing that he has chosen to leave her, and the price he is to pay is the discovery on his wedding night of a deflowered bride.

Merteuil's running narrative in her letters to Valmont as to the progress of her plans for Cécile allows Laclos to explore the physical and moral reactions of a physiologically normal, intellectually average young woman, placed in extreme circumstances. Along these lines, the novel's second letter treats the reader to an objective physical and moral description of this young virgin from the pen of the most sophisticated and attentive of observers. Merteuil informs Valmont that there are two reasons why her ex-lover Gercourt is interested in marrying this young woman: Cécile is extremely wealthy, and she is blonde. The second quality is as important as the first, for Gercourt's interest in hair color is more than a personal fancy. Merteuil explains that he believes firmly in the self-restraint of blonds (born of sexual coldness, or *la retenue*) and is counting on this lack of passion to prevent his wife from straying in the future. She finds this confidence in hair color as a sign of future fidelity ridiculous, of course; as she explains to Valmont, it is beyond question that Gercourt will end up with an unfaithful wife, but "the amusement would be in his starting off cuckolded" (14).

It is easy to forget, by the end of the novel, that Merteuil's initial plan for Cécile was merely to expedite an inevitable corruption, for letter I.2 reveals no intention of ruining the young girl completely. Merteuil's only goal is to thwart and humiliate Gercourt and to make sure that the public is informed of this embarrassment (talkative servants will fulfill this task, as outlined in letter I.63). Of more interest in this context is that Merteuil gives no reason for her apparent rejection of the theory that hair color equates to degree of sexual passion. Gercourt's opinion was physiologically sound, at least according to the humoral theory of temperament that dominated at the time of the novel's publication, for blondes were generally viewed as naturally phlegmatic and therefore more or less disinterested in sex.

It may be that Merteuil simply "knows" that all women, like all men, crave sexual activity and the resulting pleasurable sensations. Whatever the source of her dismissal of such moral indicators as hair color, Merteuil goes on in letter I.2 to describe those aspects of Cécile's overall appearance most likely to pique Valmont's interest, with her use of capital letters indicating the allegorical nature of her "tale": "The Heroine of this new Novel is worthy of all your attentions: she is truly pretty, she is only fifteen years, old; a rosebud … and has, moreover, a certain languorous expression that promises much" (14). Merteuil's use of the dismissive (and untranslatable) pronoun *cela* to refer to Cécile in place of "she" ("cela n'a que quinze ans") reveals how little she cares for the girl as a human being. Cécile is for Merteuil merely a stock fictional character type who will star in the real-life "novel" the Marquise is writing. The story line she has in mind for Cécile would no doubt follow that of the typical libertine fictions studied by Laurent Versini as possible sources for *Dangerous Liaisons*. Versini lists the character types found in such works: the clever and complicitous valet, the convent friend, the good and sensible woman, the methodical rogue, the evil couple, and—as epitomized by Merteuil, of course—"the female demon," a type he declares to be "one of the most original creations of the eighteenth-century novel."[9] As for Cécile, Versini places her under the interesting subcategory of the "false ingénue," the young girl who feigns innocence and powerlessness in order to hide the fact that she is both experienced and manipulative.

This view of Cécile, commonly accepted among critics, derives from Merteuil's development of the young girl's nature in a letter from the end of part one of the novel. Merteuil has by this time come to know Cécile somewhat better, and is astonished at what she has discovered:

> She is truly delicious! She [*cela*] has neither character nor principles; imagine how sweet and easy a companion she would be. I believe that she will never shine in terms of feeling; but everything indicates that she possesses the most extreme physical sensibility. While devoid of wit and finesse, she nevertheless has a certain natural falseness, if one can use this term, that at times astonishes even me, and that will be all the more effective in that her face offers the very image of candor and ingenuity. She is of a naturally caressing nature, and I sometimes take advantage of this to amuse myself: she becomes excited with incredible facility; and she amuses me all the more in that she knows nothing, absolutely nothing, of that which she so desires to know. Her impatience makes her so amusing; she laughs, she frets, she cries, and then she begs me to enlighten her, with a good faith that is really seductive. I am seriously almost jealous of he for whom this pleasure is reserved. (78)

---

[9]   Laurent Versini, *Laclos et la tradition* (Paris: Klincksieck, 1968), 135. For more references to the familiar topoi found in Laclos's novel, see the detailed editorial notes to *Les Liaisons dangereuses*, ed. Catriona Seth (Paris: Gallimard, 2011).

The ability to astonish Mme de Merteuil is impressive, and yet the young Cécile does so, unknowingly, by possessing a trait that the Marquise has apparently never before encountered: "a certain natural falseness, if one can say this." Merteuil's astonishment is at heart a semantic problem, for she is quite aware that "natural" and "falseness" are antithetically opposed in eighteenth-century parlance, yet she believes the two are combined in this apparently simple girl. She is wrong however, and this misreading stems from a hole in her philosophy. When Merteuil observes that Cécile's face offers the "image" of candor and ingenuity, she communicates her inability to accept that Cécile, or indeed any young girl, could be simultaneously ingenuous and sensitive to sexual stimulation. Accustomed to diagnosing all pretense to innocence as hypocrisy, Merteuil is unable to accept, fully and unequivocally, that there stands before her a young girl who is, on the one hand, completely ignorant of all matters sexual, and on the other hand, craving sexual gratification to the point of tears, at least under the influence of Merteuil's expertly licentious conversation. Merteuil accordingly decides that Cécile is a miraculously "artless" version of herself, or rather, of the social persona she has so carefully constructed: in public, an innocent, inexperienced prude; in private, a raging libertine.

In Laclos's novel, as opposed to Merteuil's novel-within-a-novel, Cécile represents not a literary type (the *fausse ingénue*), but rather a socio-cultural norm. There is nothing astonishing about her, according to the standards of the day. Her apparent "falseness" is merely the effect of her convent education coupled with her limited rational ability—the preferred "norm" for young girls. According to the latest scientific treatises, any healthy girl of Cécile's age and social status should be both brimming with sexual desire and necessarily "ignorant" of the nature of these sensations. The degree of her "truthfulness" is a moot point; she cannot be false to the principles of sexual conduct if she possesses no such "principles," indeed possesses no knowledge of the sexual nature of her sensations.

Merteuil however sees Cécile as a wondrous discovery, and as a result of her newfound appreciation for her young "friend" develops a much more elaborate plan for Mlle Volanges. In addition to exacting her revenge upon Gercourt by assuring the deflowering of his future bride, Merteuil will make this young woman her confidante, a female pendant to Valmont, or as Merteuil writes in letter II.54: "She is truly lovable, this dear young thing! ... I promised her that I would form her, and I believe I will keep my word. I have often noticed the need to have a woman in my confidence ... but I can do nothing, as long as she is not ... what she must become" (111).

Merteuil's uncharacteristically delicate ellipsis ("as long as she is not ...") is a reference to the *déniaisement* by defloration explored in Chapter 2, an operation that is now not only to rid Cécile of the virginity cherished by Gercourt but also to "enlighten" her as to the usefulness of playing the role of "false ingénue." Such knowledge must come from the (semen-filled) male of the species ("he for whom this pleasure is reserved"), but until then, and in an effort to convince Valmont to abandon his seduction of the married Présidente in favor of advancing her revenge on Gercourt, Merteuil continues to highlight Cécile's delightful physical sensibility. In the process she presents the reader with something of an eighteenth-century fictional speciality: descriptions of unwitting orgasmic pleasure experienced by a young woman. The passage occurs when Cécile boasts to the Marquise of her successful resistance to her music teacher. The young chevalier de Danceny is madly attracted to his pupil but his seduction techniques, in Merteuil's estimation, are pathetically inadequate. That Danceny's lack of technique, rather than Cécile's steadfast virtue, is to blame for his failure, is a theory that Merteuil decides to put to the test. She tells Valmont: "I, a mere woman, with words alone [*de propos à propos*], I excited her to the point where ... Well you may believe me, never was anyone so susceptible to a surprise of the senses" (111).

The most famous of such scenes is found in *The Nun*, but while Diderot's heroine Suzanne assume that she is suffering from a contagious disease when she experiences orgasm alongside her Mother Superior, Cécile does have a (very) confused idea of what is happening.[10] She writes to Sophie, her convent friend and companion in ignorance: "It seems to me that I love her [Merteuil] more as I love Danceny than as I love you; and sometimes I even wish that she were Danceny. Perhaps this is because my friendship with her is not a childhood friendship, like ours" (112). Merteuil clearly believes that Cécile's physical reaction marks her as a born libertine, but the reader is to view Cécile as merely exhibiting the degree of sensibility to be expected from any healthy young girl of her age listening to a lascivious conversation. She is both innocent and highly susceptible to sexual stimulation, having emerged from claustration a fully developed, healthy female specimen, truly the virginal "rosebud" of Merteuil's perverted medieval romance. Her "innocence" even adds greatly to her attractiveness to men, as the treatises so titillating argue, including the grasping and insipid Gercourt and the sexually jaded Valmont, but most importantly her self-chosen and (thus most appropriate) partner, the young, sensitive, and relatively innocent chevalier de Danceny.

We are to understand that the convent is not the real source of Cécile's problems, and may indeed have afforded her a brief respite from her decadent milieu. Her problem is that her mother does not take her in hand after she leaves the nuns' effective if stifling protection. Mme de Volanges, however unwittingly, hands her innocent young daughter over to the worst possible of influences, the Marquise. Another, far more telling indication that the convent is hardly the source of Cécile's eventual and spectacular fall is our knowledge, gained from the autobiographical letter II.81, that Merteuil's mother kept her at home.[11] This maternal figure is to be understood as truly vigilant in her duties, for she kept her daughter from any

---

[10] For an overview of reactions to this scene, see my "Religion in Diderot's *La Religieuse*," *XVIII New Perspectives on the Eighteenth Century* 2.1 (Spring 2005): 3–15.

[11] This autobiographical letter has elicited an impressive number of critical studies; see for example Martin Nøjgaard, "L'Education de la Marquise: Un Contre-exemple? A propos des *Liaisons dangereuses*," *Orbis Litterarum: International Review of Literary Studies* 57.6 (2002), 416–19.

knowledge of sexuality as a young girl. The Marquise tells us that she entered society, as does Cécile, quite ignorant of all things sexual. But Merteuil was never, even as a child, in any way the creation of her circumstances, at least in her own opinion; from a very young age this extraordinary woman reasoned herself into existence, she tells Valmont, deliberately choosing the principles by which she would act: "I say my principles, and I say so purposefully: for they are not, like those of other women, the result of chance, acquired with no thought and adopted by habit; they are the fruit of my profound reflections; I created them, and I can say that I am my own work" (170).

The story of her self-creation begins in full force when Merteuil's younger self is finally allowed to enter society and satisfy her considerable curiosity. The most important point that Merteuil makes in letter II.81, for my purposes, is that even prior to this coming out she was highly aware of and annoyed by her state of ignorance. She was also well aware that the adults around her were actively conspiring to keep her in the dark. She took, of course, a well-designed and effective approach to remedying this situation once she entered society. She convinced those around her of the authenticity of her unfocused stare and virtuous silence and was thus able to listen in on their whispered conversations at will: "I carefully noted that which they were attempting to hide from me" (171).

What the adults were most anxious to hide from her was any knowledge of that most interesting and forbidden of subjects, sex, referred to in letter II.81, in accordance with her youthful status at the time, as love:

> Like all young girls, I tried to understand love and its pleasures ... watched over by a vigilant mother, I had only vague ideas about love that I could not pin down; nature itself, whom I have had reason to praise ever since, was not yet giving me any signs. One might say that she was working in silence to perfect her creation. Only my head was in ferment; I did not desire to experience sexual pleasure, I wanted to know; and from the desire to learn came the knowledge of how to do so. (171–2)

The statement that only the young Merteuil's "head" was in a state of agitation is an important detail. We remember Rousseau's description of what Segrais refers to as "moral smallpox," that first sign of the coming revolution of puberty: "This stormy revolution is announced by the murmur of awakening passion: a muted fermentation warns of the approach of danger."[12] But the 14-year-old Merteuil is not "confused," withdrawn, and prone to eating bizarre substances; in other words, her mind is not "in ferment" due to the sexed genital fluids flowing from these lower organs to her brain. She is quite insistent that feelings of sexual desire did not enter into her curiosity about "love"; she felt only a burning "desire to know." Her brain, it would seem, had awakened of its own accord. This one organ, normally awakened at puberty by the influence of the genitals or at least, as in

---

[12]   Jean-Jacques Rousseau, *Emile*, in *Oeuvres complètes*, 4 vols (Paris: Gallimard, 1959–1969), IV:489–90.

Roussel's writings, in sympathy with these lower organs, already reigned supreme in this prepubescent girl.

Merteuil reads the relative tardiness of her awakening to sexual desire as a sign that nature was "working in silence to perfect her creation." This diagnosis might at first seem to have a sound physiological basis, for as explored in Chapter 2, the physiologists of puberty highlighted the benefits of such a delay, as did Rousseau in *Emile*. But while Merteuil's life is in many ways a testimony to the power of sexual desire, something else seems to be indicated here, for the hygiene treatises are quite clear that only engorgement is to awaken desire. Merteuil somehow possesses the desire to know about sex in the absence of both plethoric forces and any enlightenment as to the sex act. She knows only that something important is being carefully hidden from her, and she cannot bear to be in the dark. This type of curiosity about sex is a pure thirst for knowledge, and Laclos takes care in the passage quoted above to highlight the precise nature and source of Merteuil's curiosity: "Only my head was in ferment; I did not desire to experience sexual pleasure, I wanted to know [*je ne désirais pas de jouir, je voulais savoir*]; and from the desire to learn came the knowledge of how to do so." It is this will to know, in the absence of genital activity, that makes her a young monster. She is all the more prodigious in that only young boys, not young girls, are said to be granted intellectual clarity and strength of will at puberty, through the action of reabsorbed sperm. Even as a child, Merteuil is never, apparently, one of the hygiene treatises' mucous dominated, weak-minded creatures; she is, from birth, a reasoning machine.

An Eve with no corrupting snake (or decadent external influences) behind her thirst for knowledge, the future marquise fakes a confessional admission of perfidy in order to get information from her priest: "I accused myself of having done *everything that women do*." To her disappointment, nothing specific emerges from the resulting chastisement, although her confessor does attach so much sinfulness to whatever it is that "women do" that the young Merteuil is led to conclude that "the pleasure must be extreme; and after the desire to know, came the desire to experience." We note again that this "desire to experience" is more scientific then sensual in nature. Her willingness to wait until she is married for this experience is yet another indication of the lack of any physical component to this desire: "The certainty of knowing extinguished my curiosity, and I arrived in the arms of M. de Merteuil a virgin." This momentous night held no fears for Merteuil—although she was, of course, clever enough to fake anxiety—for she viewed losing her virginity not only as an interesting episode in her life but also as an *expérience* understood in the alternate French meaning of "experiment." She tells Valmont that she observed everything, "exactly," including the pain she felt, but that pain soon gave way to pleasure, or as she writes: "This type of study soon came to please me." That this pleasure was physical as well as intellectual in nature is indicated again later, in a statement that emphasizes Merteuil's ability to hide her feelings, in this instance from her husband: "I resolved that, given that I was highly sensitive, I would give him to believe that I was quite impassible" (172).

The power to gain knowledge from and about others is surpassed in Merteuil only by her refusal to allow others to know anything about her. No one is to have access to her thoughts, a reflex born at least in part of her feelings of powerlessness, of imposed ignorance, when she was young girl: "Only my thoughts were my own, and I was furious at the idea that someone could take them from me [*me la ravir*] against my will by force or by surprise." The obvious analogy to rape evoked by the verb *ravir* is made even more explicit in the next sentence, when Merteuil describes the techniques she developed in order to avoid being "surprised" against her will into revealing her thoughts: "Armed with these first weapons, I tried them out: no longer content merely to prevent myself from being penetrated, I enjoyed presenting myself in various guises" (171). It is her ability to remain "impenetrable" in her thoughts that gives her true power over others, and she does not lose this "virginity of the mind" until she opens herself up, at least to some degree, to Valmont, a decision that will ultimately fulfill her worst fears about her own vulnerability. When he eventually makes her letters public, this particular letter will stand out and the Marquise will pay dearly for her revelations.

While Merteuil's marriage was celebrated in an expeditious manner that gratified her desire to know, the ceremony that was to unite Gercourt with his wealthy blonde fiancée is delayed by unexpected military maneuvers. This delay allows ample time for Cécile to become ... what she must become, according to Merteuil: a young woman who in losing her physical virginity also loses her mental naiveté. The rape of Cécile occurs while she is staying at the home of the aged Mme de Rosemonde, accompanied by her mother, her mother's friend Mme de Tourvel, and Rosemonde's heir, Valmont. The Vicomte has designs on both Tourvel and Cécile, but decides to play dirty with his younger target. He obtains a copy of the key to Cécile's room by tricking Danceny into demanding it of her, and then enters while she sleeps the heavy sleep of the young and innocent.[13] He wakes her, holds her down, and threatens to blame her if she cries out for help. Turning the episode into a libertine physiology experiment, he tests what he refers to in a letter to Merteuil as the "power of the occasion" (*puissance de l'occasion*, with "occasion" another libertine topos), using just enough physical force to keep Cécile in place on her bed while he manipulates her into "voluntarily" ceding to his demands for sex: "I was mean enough to use just enough force so that she could overcome it. However, if my charming enemy tried to take advantage of my generosity by attempting to escape, I contained her by using the same fear that I had already used to such happy effect [that of waking her mother in the next room]" (213). Cécile is thus entirely sincere in her own description of this scene in a letter to Merteuil when she insists that while she had by no means wanted Valmont to continue "seducing" her, she had been unable to control her body's response to his skilled "manipulation" of her senses.

---

[13]   I have argued elsewhere for the use of "rape" to describe what is often referred to as a "seduction" ("The Rape of Cécile and the Triumph of Love in the *Liaisons dangereuses*," *Eighteenth-Century Studies* 43.1 [2009]: 1–19).

Cécile does not respond to this episode according to Merteuil's script, however. Rather than abandoning love (Danceny) in favor of sex (Valmont), she decides to lock her skilled sexual partner out of her room the next night, bolting it from the inside, despite having agreed to see him again while still under the influence of his presence. She does eventually allow Valmont back into her room after Merteuil convinces her that it will help her to unite, in time, with Danceny (yet another indication of Cécile's continuing simplicity of mind), but the Marquise is so disgusted by the young girl's loyalty to the chevalier that she abandons all hope of making her erstwhile protégée into a suitable confidante. She declares to Valmont that he is free to do with Cécile as he will: "I have become completely disinterested in her case ... she is possessed of a stupid ingenuity that did not respond even to the specific that you administered, and that never fails to work, and this, in my opinion, is the most dangerous illness that a woman can have" (244).

The use of the medical term "specific" is quite interesting here. Merteuil does not develop the theory behind her use of this term, leaving us to wonder if it is the mechanical action of opening the "womb" that is to enlighten Cécile—in accord with the iatromechanical model—or the first infusion of semen, as the humoral theory favored by the vitalists would have it. Merteuil herself, we note, required no such outside intervention by a man to awaken her to reason; she is, indeed, her own creation, as an intellectual and as a sexual creature. Whatever the details of the Marquise's diagnosis, this letter signals the end of Cécile. Merteuil decides that Gercourt will be presented on his wedding night with far more than a deflowered bride; this "pleasure machine," as Merteuil calls her, is to be transformed into a quite thoroughly debauched young woman but she is to remain absolutely ignorant of the philosophical side of libertinism.[14] She is to be made into a pitiful specimen of French womanhood, in other words, neither stupidly virtuous nor knowingly depraved. Continuing her medical analogy, Merteuil concludes her instructions to Valmont: "Have no fear in forcing the dosage ... once we have used her for our purposes, let her become what she will" (244).

It is noteworthy, in the interest of defending Cécile's physiological normality, that in spite of Merteuil's disappointment, this young girl does exhibit a strong response to her defloration, at least according to letter III.96, from the Vicomte to the Marquise. Valmont tells Merteuil that after his night in Cécile's bed he woke early, despite his nocturnal exertions, in order to observe his victim at breakfast. Or as Valmont puts it: "I passionately love to see women's expressions the day after [*les mines de lendemain*]." He describes with astonishment how physically changed Cécile is: "That face, once so very round, has become so elongated!" Even Mme de Volanges, generally unobservant, notices this physical transformation, writing to Merteuil that "in the space of several days, [my daughter] has visibly changed."

---

[14]   Michel Delon analyzes the sources and echoes of this phrase in "'Ces sortes de femmes ne sont absolument que des machines à plaisir': Les Enjeux d'une formule de Mme de Merteuil," in *Poétique de la pensée: Etudes sur l'âge classique et le siècle philosophique* (Paris: Champion, 2006), 341–51.

Misdiagnosing these symptoms as signifying a broken heart, rather than sexual initiation, Mme de Volanges momentarily wavers in her opposition to Danceny; perhaps she will, after all, allow her daughter to marry for love, rather than for status and money (Merteuil quickly puts a stop to any such notions).

But while the reader is meant to realize that Cécile's mother does indeed care deeply for her daughter, we are also to recognize that by missing the signs of sexual activity, Mme de Volanges is most of all merely failing, once again, in her motherly duties. She has obviously not read the appropriate manuals on adolescent hygiene, for it was after all in the face that girls were said to exhibit the telltale signs of sexual stimulation (parents were told to be attentive to such changes as indicative of masturbation). In her favor, Mme de Volanges is also to be understood as having neglected to read the libertine works in which such "signs" were a comic staple, as in the La Fontaine fable mentioned in Chapter 2, "Comment l'esprit vient aux filles" (1674). Evariste de Parny's poem "The Day After" ("Le Lendemain," 1778) is a more contemporary reference, in which the happy lover highlights the newly rosy cheeks and languorous eyes of his no-longer-virginal "dear Eléonore." He notes as well the "agreeable reverie" that has replaced her childish silliness, and, of particular relevance here, how Eléonore's breasts now strain against the scarf placed so carefully by motherly hands, only to be disarranged later by the hands of her lover.

None of the merely physical signs indicative of the loss of virginity interest the marquise de Merteuil, for she is looking for one precise indication that Valmont's "specific" has operated a cure, and it is absent. As the young false-ingénue heroine of the libertine novel Merteuil has been "writing," Cécile was to have experienced the "opening" of her virginal mind through intercourse. She was in other words to have been transformed into a pleasure-seeking libertine. Merteuil would have Cécile imitate such famous heroines as Thérèse of Boyer d'Argens's *Thérèse philosophe* (1748), who after merely watching Father Dirrag "minister" to the young Eradice gets down on her knees and begs God to allow her to be treated in the same way—by any man, one assumes.[15] Merteuil is convinced that the "cure" Valmont has attempted "never fails," and yet it has indeed failed, in this instance. Rather than questioning her own philosophy, and asking herself if perhaps some or even the majority of women do not work according to the physiological model in which she places her faith, Merteuil dismisses Cécile as a hopeless anomaly, just as she had (in an equally mistaken fashion) praised her earlier for personifying an oxymoron, "natural falseness."

Ultimately for the Marquise, it is love—mistaken by Cécile for a psychological reality rather than understood as a euphemism for sexual desire—that is the obstacle to this young girl's enlightenment. Cécile's persistence in believing in love after experiencing sexual fulfillment with Valmont is a fatal indictment of this

---

[15] For an analysis of philosophy in *Thérèse philosophe*, see Natania Meeker, "'I resist it no longer': Enlightened Philosophy and Feminine Compulsion in *Thérèse philosophe*," *Eighteenth-Century Studies* 39.3 (Spring 2006), 363–76.

young girl's mental potential, in Merteuil's eyes. It is no coincidence that it will be love, or rather love's frequent companion, jealousy, that ultimately destroys the Marquise, for her desire to avenge herself against Valmont's preference for Tourvel will expose her as she really is—a physical and moral monster—when Valmont makes their letters public.

Sexual Exclusivity and the Civilized Woman

In the introduction to an issue of *Yale French Studies* devoted to the topic of "Libertinage and Modernity," Catherine Cusset identifies two kinds of libertinage, a division that reflects the "degeneration" Sturm diagnoses in the phenomenon over the course of the eighteenth century. She points first to the anodyne variety of a Marivaux, a Crébillon, or a Fragonard. This kinder, gentler libertinage is characterized by the pursuit of the "surprise of the senses" (what Crébillon refers to as "the moment"), during which one is oblivious to anything but sexual pleasure. Cusset proposes that there afterward develops a second, far more active type, that of Laclos and Sade's characters, in which the manipulation of others is the ultimate goal. Both types, Cusset insists, find their opposition and therefore their definition in love. Cusset concludes, with admirable clarity and succinctness, that the message of *Dangerous Liaisons* is the following: "Laclos finally unmasks libertinage as itself a mask covering and repressing a much more powerful and truer reality: love."[16]

Determining how exactly one should define "truer" with regard to the "reality" of love in this novel will be my goal in the second part of this chapter, with the aim of exploring how the answer to this question reflects late eighteenth-century cultural presuppositions about the nature of women and of female sexuality. While Cusset finds a moral lesson in Laclos's novel ("We are superficial to the point of compromising, or losing, what is dearest to our hearts"), I see a physiological lesson, subtending moral advice that Laclos by no means believes his readers will be able to put into practice.[17] Underlying my argument is the assumption that sexuality was for Laclos a central factor determining human behavior, and that the moral value of that behavior was to be judged by the extent to which it reflected "natural" human sexuality. Laclos was, of course, far from alone in connecting innate, gendered sexuality to notions of "natural" morality, but the combination of three factors makes his case particularly representative: he wrote an essay exploring the physiology of natural puberty; he wrote a best-selling novel in which sexuality plays a central role; and he went on to be intimately involved in the politics of the French Revolution.[18]

---

[16]   Catherine Cusset, "Editor's Preface: The Lesson of Libertinage," in *Yale French Studies, Libertinage and Modernity* 94 (1998), 4.

[17]   Cusset, "Editor's Preface," 7.

[18]   In "Physicians and Philosophes: Physiology and Sexual Morality in the French Enlightenment," Kathleen Wellman observes that the connection of the physiology of

The clearest expression of Laclos's thoughts on the sexual morality of eighteenth-century French women is found in the essay mentioned above, "On Women and Their Education." Laclos's goal in this piece is to redefine women's role in French society by realigning it with natural processes, to the extent that this realignment is possible. He uses contemporary notions of the physiology of women as a tool to imagine women's sexual morality in the natural state and from there traces the fallen status of women through the first primitive social organizations up until the France of his day. Although his civilized woman exhibits many of the faults and weaknesses attributed to her by writers such as Roussel and Rousseau, his work stands out among the many treatises on women's morality published in this period in that the failings of civilized women are in no way attributable, according to his logic, to their inherent female nature, but rather to their enslavement by men, in reaction to which they must reinvent themselves in order to better their lot. Suellen Diaconoff refers to Laclos as "the first feminist writer" in France, but I am more in agreement with Liselotte Steinbrügge's reading: "Laclos is primarily concerned not with liberating women from patriarchal chains but with demonstrating the general decay afflicting society. Woman is the chief victim of this development."[19]

Steinbrügge adds that women are the most visible symptoms of this decline in Laclos, a point not unique to his work, of course, but present in many of the treatises I have been examining in this study. What is unusual about Laclos, if not unique, is that he specifically addresses his women readers, and does so while addressing the topic of sexual pleasure and promiscuity. He invites women to consider the advantages that their free, strong foremothers enjoyed in the state of nature and lost only when organized society began to develop. The goal of his essay, he tells us, is to indicate to women "the road that they are to take to find themselves again" (391). They will be going backward down this road, for he is proposing a negative education, in the sense that he wants to help women to unlearn what their society has taught them. That an active, positive education would be an impossibility is made clear in an earlier, unfinished essay that reveals the fundamentally dark view Laclos takes of woman's chances in civilized society in general, a vision more than adequately represented in his novel as well: "Wherever there is slavery, there can be no education; in every society, women are slaves; therefore, woman in society is uneducable."[20]

The scientific basis of Laclos's argument relies on assumptions that are never clearly stated, but that obviously reflect those of the physiological treatises of the period, and to a certain extent the natural histories of the period as well. Laurent Versini has pointed out that the expressions Laclos uses in "On Women"

sex to morality is common in both physiological and philosophical writings from the Enlightenment (*Eighteenth-Century Studies* 35.2 [Winter 2002], 267).

[19] Suellen Diaconoff, "Resistance and Retreat: A Laclosian Primer for Women," *University of Toronto Quarterly* 38.3 (1989); Liselotte Steinbrügge, *The Moral Sex: Woman's Nature in the French Enlightenment* (New York: Oxford University Press, 1995), 88.

[20] Choderlos de Laclos, "Discours," in *Oeuvres complètes*, 391.

to describe the progression from childhood to adulthood of his "natural girl" are nearly identical to those given by Buffon in "A Natural History of Man."[21] As Versini points out, Laclos even reproduces the chapter titles of this section of Buffon's *Natural History*: "On Childhood," "On Puberty," "On Adulthood," and "On Old Age and Death." Laclos's "On Women and Their Education" might indeed have been given the title "A Natural History of Woman," for Laclos devotes the greater part of this essay to describing woman's sexuality in the state of nature, a rather neglected subtopic within the many eighteenth-century descriptions of this primordial state available to him.

This lack of interest in specifically female human sexuality in the so-called "state of nature" reflects the relative neglect of a young girl found in 1731 living "wild" in the Champagne region of France. As Julia Douthwaite has observed, this "wild child," afterwards christened Marie-Angélique Leblanc, was by no means as famous as her male counterparts Peter of Hanover (found in 1725) or Victor of Aveyron (1797).[22] While Marie-Angélique was the object of extraordinary stories concerning her physical prowess and avidity for raw meat, as well as her violent reactions to being touched, especially by men, Douthwaite notes that Marie-Angélique had far fewer visitors than Peter or Victor and that, more notably, she was excluded from the type of training to which they were subjected, intended to "rationalize" the young men. She was rather, in accordance with the feminine ideal of the time, trained to be a "virtuous" woman and indeed spent the better part of her adult life in a convent. While Laclos never mentions Marie-Angélique, Buffon refers to her in passing in his *Natural History*, (quite reasonably) observing that neither she nor Peter, her close contemporary, can be said to represent human life in the state of nature. For Buffon, these two had obviously "been born into human society and no doubt abandoned in the woods, not as babies, for they would have perished, but at four, five, or six years of age."[23] Life in the state of nature is rather consistent with that of present-day "savage tribes," Buffon declares.

Laclos's principal point of reference is neither wild children nor "savage" tribes, however, but rather the theoretical treatments of human life in the state of nature that were common during this period. He of course cites the most famous of these works, Rousseau's *Discourse on the Origin and Foundation of Inequality among Men* (393, note).[24] As Laclos is, even more strongly than Rousseau, arguing for the positive advantages of the state of nature, he pauses to consider attacks on the desirability of this stage of human development, limiting himself, as he notes,

---

[21]   Laclos, *Oeuvres complètes*, 1426, note 2.

[22]   Julia Douthwaite, *The Wild Girl, Natural Man, and the Monster* (Chicago: University of Chicago Press, 2002).

[23]   George-Louis Leclerc, comte de Buffon, *Histoire naturelle, générale et particulière*, 36 vols. (Paris: Imprimerie Royale, 1749–1788), VII:29–30. Douthwaite considers Buffon's views of wild children in *The Wild Girl*, 27–8.

[24]   For an analysis of Laclos's essay in relation to Rousseau's views, see Steinbrügge, *The Moral Sex*, 83–9.

to those of Voltaire and Buffon (the latter was not impressed with what he had read about the life of "savage" tribesmen).[25] Laclos supports Rousseau's argument, in contradiction of both these influential thinkers, for the essentially solitary nature of human beings in the state of nature, then goes on to add significantly to the limited emotional range allotted to natural man by Rousseau: "His sensitive soul knows pity and love; his mind is enlightened as to his needs" (412). Just as the addition of pity to Thomas Hobbes's brutish and violent model of natural man from the *Leviathan* (1651) was one of Rousseau's central points, the positing of love as an element of "natural" existence—of natural sexuality—is crucial to an understanding of Laclos's natural woman.[26]

Laclos's insistence that natural man knows love is a contradiction of Rousseau's phylogenetic account of human society, for in the *Discourse*, this passion appears only at the moment when small groups of men and women first band together. These small tribes constitute the "second stage" of natural existence for Rousseau, still devoid of laws and the concept of ownership but no longer solitary. For Laclos, the ability to experience this most heady and profound of emotions is instead a central component of sexuality in the state of nature. Rather than the appearance of love, it is the prolongation of this powerful emotion past the moment of physical satiety that differentiates the civilized from the natural sex act. Natural man and natural woman are instead fully promiscuous, for there is nothing to prompt them to stay together after they have satisfied their strong sexual urges. Their "love" is as fleeting as the pleasure they experience, and indissolubly linked to it.

These tenets of natural sexuality are established by Laclos in the course of his lengthy narration of a prototypical natural girl's coming to sexuality. We are presented first with a young, decidedly prepubescent individual, who is both physically and morally at the opposite extreme of her enervated, eighteenth-century, urban-dwelling counterpart. Our natural girl is well fed and physically active and her skin is bronzed by exposure to the sun, traits that translate in the moral realm into complete protection from the one lascivious influence she may encounter as she goes through her day's activities: the sight of passionately coupling pairs. We are told that should natural girl come upon such a scene, she will continue on indifferently, without blushing, without fleeing, without so much as a furtive backward glance. She will above all not feel aroused, nor even curious, for she sees these acts with "the body's eyes, not the soul's; her senses are still asleep; they wait for the cry of nature to awaken them" (399). "The soul's eyes" are of course those of the imagination, for Laclos goes on to attribute the current

---

[25]   See Buffon, *Histoire naturelle*, VII:25–31.

[26]   While Thomas Kavanagh labels love in Laclos an imaginary concept, I see love as an essential element of sexual desire in Laclos's natural state, however short-lived, and thus not a complete illusion in the state of civilization (Kavanagh, "Educating Women: Laclos and the Conduct of Sexuality," in *The Ideology of Conduct: Essays on Literature and the History of Sexuality*, ed. Nancy Armstrong and Leonard Tennenhouse [New York: Methuen, 1987], 153).

degenerate state of the human race to untimely puberty brought on by "the fire of the imagination which, in society, almost never fails to be set alight" (399). In making this point, Laclos evokes the superior moral rectitude and physical power of the Gaulish ancestors of the eighteenth-century French, as do so many of the cultural theorists of decadence: "The degenerate men of today would have us believe that the monumental strength attributed to our forefathers is merely a novelistic fantasy" (399).

Despite Laclos's attacks on the notion that man is a social being by nature, his young girl is not one of Rousseau's truly solitary wanderers. We are never told the details of her life—where she sleeps or how she spends the majority of her time—but we are told that her kind group together to hunt, and for other, unnamed events. On one such occasion, her hand accidentally touches the hand of a young man, and she blushes. The emotion behind this blush is important; we are told that she is not ashamed—does not blush out of modesty (*pudeur*)—but is rather aroused, confusedly so, for she of course has no knowledge of what this strong physical sensation means. Unbeknownst to her, although not to the informed eighteenth-century reader, our natural girl is experiencing an early symptom of "nature's call." Her vital "interior forces" are about to come fully into play. We know that these forces have been silently at work within her by the exterior changes said to have preceded this arousal: increasing roundness, budding breasts, and the appearance of hair on her "generative parts" (400).

Natural girl withdraws to adjust to this strange new feeling, which quickly develops into a primordial version of the "mental smallpox" cited in Chapter 1. In a prelinguistic, presocietal state, this turmoil consists merely of a vague sense of ennui and unease. She simultaneously begins to experience many uncomfortable physical symptoms, all in accord with the hygiene treatises as well as with Buffon's description of puberty: a slight swelling of the groin area, headaches, and, most importantly, "all the signs of plenitude," especially swollen breasts and genitals. Menstruation soon arrives to disperse these uncomfortable symptoms, but the relief provided by this expulsion of excess fluids in the form of blood is only temporary. A new "problem" surfaces, but not immediately, of course; for sexual desire in its full-blown form will appear only after this young natural girl's womb (or "nature's laboratory," as Laclos calls it) has had time to prepare for childbirth. Only after she is completely prepared for childbirth does the young natural woman, as she has now become, begin to experience the full force of natural sexual desire, "a devouring fire lit by nature, and that pleasure alone will extinguish" (400–401).

We note that the protection from members of the opposite sex necessary to this interlude between first menstruation and the full development of the womb is provided for by nature in this young girl's case. She feels the instinctual urge to seek a solitary hiding place when the first troubling feelings of puberty are born within her, and stays there until this process has run its course. While societies of all kinds, we are to understand, must provide a temporary "prison" for their adolescent girls, be it Cécile's convent or the white veils and chains Diderot attributes to the Tahitians, in the Laclosian state of nature the young girl is protected from premature sexual activity and childbirth by the instinct to remove herself from the society of men until she is fully ready for sex. But while the hygiene treatises recommend that parents allow at least two years between the onset of menses and marriage in girls, Laclos tells his readers that natural girl's solitary self-confinement is far shorter. Less time is needed between first menstruation and procreation in the natural state, for puberty is never premature in nature, but occurs only when the body is fully developed and ready (399). This young girl's brain is also awakened by natural puberty, a sign that her mind well as her body is in the process of becoming fully adult. These new intellectual faculties manifest themselves in a young girl living in the state of nature as a sudden appreciation for the beauties of the natural world, all of which work together in turn to enhance her sensual feelings. The perfume of flowers increases her feelings of voluptuousness, and bird song is no longer mere background noise, but a harmony that "speaks to her heart."

The young girl's ever increasing sexual drive reaches both crisis and resolution at dawn. She has not slept, and her vain attempts to quench her "fire" in the river have left her burning still: "It is then, at a distance, that she perceives a man; a powerful instinct, an involuntary movement, makes her run to him; as she draws closer, she becomes timid, she stops; but, carried away once more, she goes to him and takes him in her arms ... Delicious pleasure [*jouissance*], who would dare try to describe you?" (401).

At this point, Laclos tells us, his natural woman has "reached the point of perfection; she can only fall from now on [*déchoir*]." He adds: "Before she begins to experience nature's abandonment, let us stop a moment and consider her" (402). She most evidently possesses three positive qualities: freedom, strength, and health. But what of those other two qualities so prized by women, "beauty and love"? She is beautiful, but we must judge her as one would judge country "fruit," rather than the products of a hothouse, we are told. As for love, the answer is quite precise: "We agree that there could be no continuing passion between two beings who join together never having seen each other before, and soon separate, never to see each other again. But this moment is not indivisible and, if we examine it closely, we are able to perceive all the nuances of sentiment" (403). Laclos traces the exact correlations between the course of natural and civilized sex acts, with the natural couple's first caresses taking the place of the civilized couple's "declaration of love." The natural lovers are even said to be able to communicate the depth of their feelings to each other, not by elegant phrases, of course, but with "humid looks" and "burning sighs." The main difference between these primordial lovers and ourselves, Laclos harshly declares, is that "[they] leave each other without distaste" (403).

In most details (other than the inclusion of "love") Laclos's description of natural sexuality is perfectly standard for his era. There is nothing new for example in his emphasis on the burning intensity of natural woman's sexual desire, nor in his attributing the sexual initiative to this young woman. Her sudden timidity when she draws close to her partner is also standard (although most writers have her flee in mock resistance). There were of course, as always, exceptions to this view of female sexuality; Antoine-Léonard Thomas, in his *Essay on Women*, has women possess only a "timid desire": "For nature gave to one of the two sexes the audacity of desire and the right to attack, to the other defense and that timid desire that attracts by resisting. Love is for the one sex a conquest, and for the other a sacrifice."[27] In his review of Thomas's work for Grimm's *Literary Correspondence* (1772), a piece that became an essay on women in its own right, Diderot goes so far as to deny women much sexual feeling at all. He declares their orgasms rare or perhaps even altogether absent: "The highest happiness flees from them even in the arms of the man they adore," while men, he declares, can find this "sovereign happiness" with any willing woman. The reason for this difference is of course said to be physiological, and connected to the "delicate female organs" mentioned by both Thomas and Diderot: "Organized in the opposite manner of ourselves, the mechanism [*mobile*] in women that gives rise to [*sollicite*] voluptuousness is so delicate, and its source is so far removed, that it is not extraordinary for it never to arrive or to lose its way." We are to understand that the source of women's sexual desire is her active imagination, or her heart; while in men this source is, as Diderot refers to it, "a more indulgent organ."[28]

While Laclos does not contradict the majority of commentators in postulating a high degree of sexual feeling in his natural woman, he does differ radically in the tender and appealing tone with which he writes about the resulting advances she makes on a man. *Gulliver's Travels into Several Remote Nations of the World* (1726) contains one of the best-known negative representations of lustful natural women, in the form of the female Yahoos. Jonathan Swift's novel appeared in a French translation in 1727 and went through a number of editions. Swift's eighteenth-century French readers would have encountered the Yahoos, a degenerate race of human being, in the last section of the novel, when Gulliver begins to write about his stay among yet another strange race, the equine Houyhnhnms, a term that roughly translates (from horse language) as "the perfection of nature." By the time that Gulliver is the object of a particularly enthusiastic display of "natural" female desire on the part of a Yahoo, he has been so inculcated with the cerebral and refined Houyhnhnm culture that the shock is strong and lasting. Upon his (forced) return to England, he cannot bear the presence of his wife; indeed, the knowledge that he had copulated with her and produced children leaves poor Gulliver thoroughly nauseated.

So beastly are the Yahoos that Gulliver does not at first recognize his kinship with them, although the ruling horses are able to identify Gulliver as a Yahoo, albeit far paler and much less hirsute (his clothing gives them pause as well). They also note his very short claws and his "affectation of walking continually

---

[27]   Antoine-Léonard Thomas, *Essai sur le caractère, les moeurs, et l'esprit des femmes dans les différents siècles* (Paris: Champion, 1987), 46.

[28]   Denis Diderot, "Sur les femmes," in *Oeuvres* (Paris: Gallimard, 1951), 950.

on [his] two hinder feet."[29] The Yahoos immediately recognize Gulliver as one of their own, as proved by the attraction the female Yahoos evidence for him. Yahoo sex is very much driven by female lust, for as we learn from Gulliver's equine Master, the females hide behind bushes waiting for a male Yahoo, then jump out and employ "antick Gestures and Grimaces" to attract his attention. Should the male advance, the female will then "slowly retire, looking often back, and with a counterfeit Show of Fear, run off into some convenient Place" (245). Gulliver comments: "I could not reflect without some Amazement, and much Sorrow, that the Rudiments of *Lewdness*, *Coquetry*, *Censure*, and *Scandal*, should have Place by Instinct in Womankind" (246).

Gulliver's horror is doubled when he himself becomes the object of attention of one of these females, a notably young Yahoo, for he estimates her age to be 11, making her puberty quite precocious by eighteenth-century standards. He tells us that he had been briefly separated from his Houyhnhnm guard, having stripped "stark naked" to bathe himself in a cool river, when a "young Female *Yahoo* standing behind a Bank, saw the whole Proceeding; and inflamed by Desire, as the Nag and I conjectured, came running with all Speed, and leaped into the Water within five Yards of the Place where I bathed" (248). We are told that she embraced Gulliver in a "most fulsome manner" and only reluctantly "quitted her Grasp" upon the arrival of the horse, whereupon she stood upon the bank "gazing and howling all the time I was putting on my Cloaths" (249). He declares himself to have never in his life been so afraid.

In her reading of this episode from a postcolonial perspective, Pamela Cheek notes the existence of sexual desire as a means of species identification, but concludes that Gulliver's disgust with his wife upon returning home is the result of his "colonization" by the horses, who convince him of "his own essential abjection or lack of humanity."[30] I would argue for a different or perhaps additional role that the colonial experience plays in this novel, involving the configuration of the highly complex "humanity" of the Yahoos. These creatures are not to be understood as "natural" in the sense of primordial, for they are rather a degenerate form of the human species. We learn all this when, after the horses have convinced Gulliver that he is indeed of the same "race" as the Yahoos, our hero attempts to "account for their degenerate and brutal nature" (222). His Master reveals that these creatures are not *Ylnhniamshy* (Aborigines of the Land), for according to Houyhnhnm legend, "many Ages ago, two of these Brutes appeared together upon a Mountain." Removed from their native habitat, or climate—having somehow wandered into a metaphorical land in which the atmosphere produces a highly rational race of horses that follow all the dictates of nature—these errant human travelers degenerated by degrees, and "became in

---

[29]   Jonathan Swift, *Gulliver's Travels* (Oxford: Oxford University Press, 2008), 221. Future references in the text.

[30]   Pamela Cheek, *Sexual Antipodes: Enlightenment Globalization and the Placing of Sex* (Stanford: Stanford University Press, 2003), 132.

the Process of Time, much more savage than those of their own Species in the Country whence the two Originals came" (253).

Gulliver is the object of Swift's satirical talents as well, of course, for having become so "purified" of human passions during his time with the Houyhnhnms that he is unable to bear the presence of his wife and children. The most severely treated creatures in this section of Swift's novel are however the Yahoo women, and by extension their European sisters. The sexual desires of European women, we are to understand, are held in check by social restraints so feeble that they cannot withstand a change of climate. Their "virtuous" modesty is born of a sadly lewd, counterfeit show of fear.

This same view is present in the (far gentler) works of eighteenth-century physiologists, for these writers present the attempt to repress female sexual desire as the cause of the worst excesses in women. This vision of female sexuality is perhaps most explicitly described in the *Encyclopédie* article "Satyriasis" (1765), by Ménuret de Chambaud. Although satyriasis or priapism is attributed exclusively to men, women are said to be likewise subject to "diseases that are characterized by an insatiable desire for venereal pleasures":

> Illnesses of this type act more quickly in women, and are much more aggressive; already more lively than men's, women's imaginations are altered by the constraint imposed upon them by the rules of behavior they have been taught; this restraint worsens the effects [of the disease], and soon drives these unfortunates to the brink of insanity; then, under the empire of the disease and hearing only the voice of nature, they seek to obey it; they no longer know decency or modesty; nothing seems shameful to them as long as it works to satisfy their desires; they harass all men indifferently, throwing themselves wildly into their arms, or attempt by means indicated by nature but proscribed by virtue to supplement the lack of men.[31]

As pointed out in Chapter 1, Ménuret de Chambaud was exceptional in having, however implicitly, argued for masturbation as a possible cure for some sexual disorders, including satyriasis. Of more interest to me here is the implied liveliness of the sexuality of women who listen "only to the voice of nature." Ménuret equates, in other words, the sexuality of "natural" women with that of "diseased" civilized women. Quite obviously, in Ménuret's view as in that of many others, "natural" female sexuality is hardly an ideal to be sought after by contemporary women.

Such is the case as well in one of the articles to which Ménuret refers us, "Uterine Furor" (1757) by Arnulphe d'Aumont. A doctor, d'Aumont contributed a great number of articles to the *Encyclopédie*, covering a wide variety of medical topics, including one of great interest to this study, "Childhood," in which he emphasizes the importance of hygiene as a tool for temperament formation.

---

[31] "Satyriasis," in *Encyclopédie, ou Dictionnaire raisonné des sciences, des arts et des métiers*, ed. Denis Diderot and Jean d'Alembert (Paris: Briasson [etc.], 1751–1765), XIV:703.

In "Uterine Furor," we are told that if men exhibited sexual desire as intense as that of women suffering from this disease, it would be termed "venereal furor." But men never do; for one thing, they are not subjected to the same laws of conduct as are women, and thus never reach the degree of "delirium" demonstrated by nymphomaniacal women. D'Aumont then moves on, apparently forgetting this repression hypothesis, and points out that the moral causes of excessive desire—the list includes the usual suspects: licentious conversations, etc.—are common to both sexes, and thus cannot account for the observation that this particularly virulent form of venereal furor occurs only in women. The answer for this disparity is therefore said to be found in the specific physical conformation of the female sex. Uterine furor can be brought on by plethoric pressure during menstruation, an excitement that does not dissipate when the flow is blocked. Or it may be caused by an overabundance of the "salivary humor" (phlegm) in the glands of the vagina, said to irritate the excretory vessels in a manner similar to menstrual plethora. The presence of "phlegm" in the vagina and its supposedly "irritating" (stimulating) quality take us back to the realm of "white flowers," as discussed in Chapter 2.

Climate plays a role in female sexual desire as well, of course, with the most dramatic example of environmentally determined female lust found in Rousseau's *Emile*. At the beginning of Book Five, "Sophie," the tutor conjectures that there might somewhere be a country subject to climatic conditions such that natural female coquetry does not exist. This place would have such a hot, inflaming atmosphere the men would easily become the victims of their Bacchic female counterparts. Despite their inherent physical superiority, these men would be "dragged to their deaths without being able to defend themselves."[32] The tutor leaves this example in the realm of speculation, for the assumption of innate female "modesty" is yet another firmly held eighteenth-century belief concerning natural sexuality, demonstrated even by Swift's female Yahoos with their "counterfeit Show of Fear." Diderot uses a Biblical metaphor in "On Women," declaring that women always and everywhere are provided with "a fig leaf, inherited from their first ancestor." He parodies the education given to eighteenth-century French girls by telling us that a mother's sole concern is to teach her daughter how to wear this fig leaf properly: "My daughter, take care of your fig leaf; your fig leaf is doing well, your fig leaf is not doing well."[33]

Liselotte Steinbrügge notes the importance of modesty to the eighteenth-century conception of woman as the "moral sex": "The female sense of modesty—half natural drive, half 'civilized' feeling—is the main determinant of female virtuousness … Man contains his passions through his capacity for reason, woman with the help of her *feeling* of modesty … Woman's depravation is the depravation of her modesty (*pudeur*)."[34] Laclos's brief nod toward innate female modesty in his description of his natural girl's first sexual experience is made more explicit

---

[32] Rousseau, *Emile*, 694.
[33] Diderot, "Sur les femmes," 957.
[34] Steinbrügge, *The Moral Sex*, 68.

in a later passage on the state of nature in which he refers to women who "by turns flee and provoke" their partners (403). That such behavior is instinctual and yet no barrier to natural woman's enthusiasm for multiple partners is essential to understanding Laclos's history of sexuality. Most importantly, women are not assigned any responsibility for the initial appearance of monogamy. We are told (in a nod to Rousseau) that after inventing the notion of property, men decided that they want to include a woman among their possessions. We are not yet witnessing the development of postcoital love; men are merely, by virtue of their superior strength, able to claim the weaker sex as their own. They use "their" women as slaves to do the less desirable work, while they go off and hunt.

This vision of woman's role in "savage" societies was quite common. In his *Sketch for a Historical Tableau of the Progress of the Human Mind* (1793–1794), for example, Condorcet includes among the drawbacks of the first stage of human society—defined, as usual, as life in small groups—a treatment of women that condemns them to a sort of slavery.[35] In his *Essay on Women*, Antoine-Léonard Thomas similarly observes that "more than half of the globe is covered with savages; and the women of all of these peoples are very unhappy."[36] In sharp contrast to Laclos, however, Thomas does not see the development of society as creating women's enslavement but rather as the means to decrease it by "softening" the savage mores of men. Fortunately for French women, this development is climate based and they enjoy a temperate climate in which attenuated (male) desire, Thomas tells us, allows for women's freedom.

While Diderot chides Thomas for dwelling on the material aspects of women's fate rather than "dipping his pen in a rainbow" and emphasizing their mysterious charms, his own essay contains a view of women's physical existence that is truly terrifying. We are told that while young girls are, like young boys, subject to all the illnesses of childhood, they are also neglected and given no education. Worse yet, they are said to suffer all too soon from:

> ... the illness that prepares them to become wives and mothers: and at that time [they] become sad, nervous, melancholic, to the alarm of their parents, worried not only for the health and the life of their child, but even more for her character: for it is at this critical moment that a young girl becomes that which she will remain her entire life, clever or stupid, sad or happy, serious or lighthearted, good or bad, the hopes of her mother dashed or realized.[37]

Puberty, as the authors of the hygiene treatises specify, both brings on an initial period of morosity and then fixes a child's temperament, for better or worse; but Diderot's description leaves little room for the hope expressed in the treatises concerning the possibilities of hygiene theory.

---

[35]   Jean-Antoine-Nicolas de Caritat, marquis de Condorcet, *Esquisse d'un tableau historique des progrès de l'esprit humain* (Paris: Vrin, 1970), 51.

[36]   Thomas, *Essai*, 1.

[37]   Diderot, *Sur les femmes*, 954.

Laclos does present the condition of women in more highly "civilized" societies as an improvement over that of "savage" women living in small communities, but he credits women's cleverness in manipulating men for this improvement. The source of this ingenuity is necessity: women's mental capacities are brought to full fruition by their harsh situation in nascent societies. It is important to note as well that this manipulation is made possible only by a secondary outgrowth of the notion of property: monogamy and the association of physical with moral properties made possible by this long-term relationship:

> As soon as society, in which the work of nature is constantly transformed, had changed the fleeting union of the sexes into a lasting liaison, pleasurable sensations ceased to be the only tie between them. Moral qualities began to be prized, and from that moment, the exterior signs of these qualities became part of what constituted beauty in the eyes of those seeking them. (427)

Laclos goes on to explain that the men of each civilization, as it advances, perceive this relationship between "beauty" and "morality" in a unique manner, suited to their vices and virtues. As had so many commentators before him, Laclos proposes a scale of national morality based on each society's women: "An attentive observer could judge the mores of each nation by [its women], with perhaps more exactitude than historians" (428). The physical aspects of these women become by this system of judgment so many signs of this varying social morality, and Laclos cites a number of messages attached to various differences in female physiognomy. Each is designed to appeal to a different variety of masculine desire, in accordance with the mores of the woman's society: I am an easy conquest; I am totally submissive to you; I possess a charming languor, or to the contrary, a lively sensibility; I possess wit, grace, talents, enough to make you overlook my lack of physical beauty. The French are said to prefer, of course, vivacity and a woman's capacity to feel pleasure, while the Swiss and the English are said to prefer sweetness and modesty. Laclos notes that while the statues of ancient Roman women reveal that their men appreciated a companion with an enthusiastic love of liberty, these sculptures also reveal women possessed of greatness of soul and a severe sense of virtue.

Laclos and Thomas's view of women as the victims of male repression was not the only story told in the eighteenth century, needless to say. Rousseau, famously, denounces the "moral aspect" of love as wholly the invention of women, part of their scheme to overturn nature by turning the masters into slaves.[38] While Laclos of course views women as the slaves of men rather than as the controlling puppet masters in all this, he does place one, originary "sin" to woman's account, for he conjures up a secular Eve: "Be it by force or by persuasion, the first woman who ceded [to monogamy] forged the chains of her entire sex" (420). We are reminded, perhaps intentionally, of yet another famous passage from the *Discourse on Inequality*, in which Rousseau places the blame for poverty on the acquiescence

---

[38] Jean-Jacques Rousseau, *Discours sur l'origine de l'inégalité*, in *Oeuvres complètes*, III:158.

by long-ago ancestors to the first man who placed markers around a plot and declared it his own. Laclos's reference to forged chains echoes yet another text by Rousseau on loss of freedom, the 1762 *Social Contract*: born free, women are everywhere, as Laclos presents them, enchained.

Like Rousseau's suffering poor, Laclos's enslaved women are oppressed by a false state of affairs that they do not recognize as such. Teaching them the complex historical reality behind their situation, so that they may act to improve their lot, is the goal of his essay, although precisely which "road" women are to take in order to "find themselves again" is not indicated until the twelfth and last chapter of this essay, "On Adornment." Given that women need protectors in civilized societies, Laclos will teach them how best to "fix" a man to them. But despite his title, Laclos does not give makeup and wardrobe tricks, such as those found in *Abdeker: Or the Art of Preserving Beauty* (1754). Written by Antoine Le Camus, regent of the Paris Medical School, the work is attributed to a court physician and purports to contain his cosmetic recipes, designed to help the Sultan's favorite cover her blushings when she is in the presence of both her lover and the Sultan's spies.

As Tassie Gwilliam notes, there is a definite element of feminocentrism at the heart of this work: "By presenting the stabilization of a woman's complexion as a hedge against unjust sexual surveillance, *Abdeker* justifies feminine disguise, removing the woman from the prying eyes of patriarchal authority and returning her to a world of private and personal sexuality."[39] Women are still, Gwilliam notes, confined to the arena of the "private and personal" in *Abdeker*, and Laclos's essay is ultimately more confining, for he would have women avoid "disguise" or risk losing their male protectors. Laclos tells women that they must ensure above all that the messages their dress and facial expressions are sending correspond to an interior reality. In contrast to the court physician Abdeker, he would have women adjust their emotions, rather than their cosmetics: "You must not be content merely to regulate your actions, you must also master the states of your soul; there are feelings that destroy beauty; if you do not repress frequent accesses of anger, your muscles will acquire a dangerous mobility, and soon all of your expressions will be grimaces" (431). If one would attach a man, one must not only appear morally worthy, one must incarnate moral worthiness—the specifics of which are left undefined, although we imagine them to be sweetness, fidelity, agreeableness, and so on. From the splendid freedom enjoyed by Laclos's natural girl we have returned to the "new woman" of the hygiene treatises, gentle and soft, revealing all her humors through the thin, white skin of her face and breasts.

Merteuil works strenuously to convince Valmont that Tourvel is nothing more than a run-of-the-mill prude whose blushes reveal her hypocrisy and limited imagination, but the reader is to recognize Tourvel as that rare civilized specimen of the female sex whose outward appearance is in absolute accord with

---

[39]   Tassie Gwilliam, "Cosmetic Poetics: Coloring Faces in the Eighteenth Century," in *Body and Text in the Eighteenth Century* (Stanford: Stanford University Press, 1994), 145.

her highly virtuous interior. She is, in other words, in agreement with Laclos's later admonitions to women. Valmont writes to Merteuil (sealing his fate in the process):

> Her face, you say, is devoid of expression. And what would she express, at those moments when her heart is silent? No, without a doubt, she does not possess, like our coquettes, that lying look that at times seduces and always fools us. She does not know how to cover the emptiness of a sentence with a studied smile; and, although she has the most beautiful teeth in the world, she laughs only when she is amused by something ... at the slightest praise or teasing word, the touching embarrassment of an unfeigned modesty paints itself on her celestial face! (21)

That this ideal exists, by some miracle, in the corrupt society of the eighteenth-century French upper classes is meant to evoke yet another impossibly virtuous fictional creation—although in an ironic allusion to Rousseau's novel, Tourvel's lady's maid, Julie, is easily seduced by Valmont's valet into revealing her mistress's habits.

As a result of her transparency, Tourvel achieves the seemingly impossible feat of "fixing" the most legendary of roués, Valmont. Not that he ceases to have sex with other women, needless to say, but he does experience with Tourvel the highly "civilized" experience of continuing to feel emotion after his physical desire has been satisfied. Their first sexual act serves merely to make her Valmont's conquest; she is in fact unconscious during his "triumph," an echo, perhaps, of Julie's swoon when she first kisses Saint-Preux, and of her "languorous" lovemaking. It is of the second union, which follows immediately, that Valmont declares: "It was with this naïve or sublime candor that she gave over to me her person and her charms, and increased my happiness by sharing it. Our fervor was complete and reciprocal; and for the first time, my own survived the culmination of my pleasure" (295). He ranks her among the "types" of women he delineates as one of the most rare, indeed, unique in his experience: "a delicate and sensitive woman, totally devoted to love, and who saw in love only her lover; whose emotions, far from taking the ordinary route, departed from her heart, only then arriving at her senses" (310). Still mistaking his love for libertine experimentation, he declares that having sought her out for "observation," he will linger with her a bit longer to complete his "work."

This type of woman—one who mistakes love for her lover—is precisely the most insipid, in Merteuil's estimation: "truly superstitious, they have for the Priest the respect and the faith that is due only to the Divinity" (170). While Valmont's delusion that he is still operating in the libertine register as a "researcher" is more than obvious to Merteuil, she recognizes the danger to Valmont and tells him that he has—most embarrassingly for a libertine—fallen in love. More importantly, Merteuil also recognizes the insult to herself, and uses Valmont's resistance to accept his situation to avenge herself by having him write a truly unforgivable letter to Tourvel. Merteuil strikes so well at the Présidente's heart that the latter exercises the only option open to her as a superior moral being: she wills herself to die, à la Clarissa Harlowe, retiring to the convent where she was educated.[40] Convents do represent, if nothing else, a useful locus of feminine withdrawal from society in this novel; Cécile similarly retreats after she realizes that she and Danceny will never be united.

Merteuil's project of ridding herself of a rival begins with a declaration, however tepid, of her own love for Valmont: "During the period when we loved each other, for I do believe that it was love, I was happy" (306–7). It is entirely possible to read in this use of a term she had previously reviled an effort to trick Valmont, as does Laurent Versini in an editorial note to this letter: "Mme de Merteuil is thinking only of once again placing her chains on Valmont, by usurping the language that gives value to her rival" (1366). But this same letter has already offered us an interesting and complex dissertation on the nature of love, one that cannot be so easily dismissed as merely manipulative:

> Have you not yet noticed that pleasure, which is in effect the sole motive for the coming together of the two sexes, does not suffice to form a liaison between them? and that if it is preceded by the desire that brings them together, it is nonetheless followed by a distaste that repels? It is a law of nature that varies only in the presence of love; and love, does one possess it when one wishes? It is however always necessary; and this would make for great difficulties, if one were not to notice that fortunately only one partner is required to love. This makes things only half as difficult, and calls for no great sacrifice; for in this situation, the one partner has the pleasure of loving, and the other of being found pleasing, less intense it is true, but when joined to the pleasure of deception, it balances out; and all is well. (305)

The Marquise, in other words, understands that an emotional attachment to one's partner may persist after the sex act, and that this prolongation is an important, even essential factor in relationships among civilized men and women, for whom the "laws of nature" no longer entirely hold true. The libertine retains power by being always the loved one, never the one who loves; and although this position entails a loss in degree of pleasure, this loss is, for Merteuil, made up for by the pleasure one feels in the mastery of deceiving one's lover. Such power is all important to her—unless we believe that the love she feels for Valmont, who obviously prefers Tourvel, has turned the tables on her at last.

While resolving the issue of Merteuil's feelings and motives is ultimately impossible—she ends her letter: "But tell me, Vicomte, which one of us will take on the task of deceiving the other?"—Laclos has already provided us with a guide to reading this critical missive, for it is placed just after an epistolary treatise on the same subject by an undoubtedly sincere source,

---

[40]   On Tourvel's death as integral to her moral outlook, see Marie Wellington, "Dying for Love? Three Case Studies: Prévost, Voltaire, Laclos," *Dalhousie French Studies* 45 (Winter 1998): 3–17.

Mme de Rosemonde (letter IV.130).[41] The importance of this missive is also made clear in Laclos's response to a letter from Marie-Jeanne Riccoboni. This famous older novelist had complained that Merteuil is both unrealistically evil and will give foreigners a false idea of French women. In defending his creation, Laclos cites letter IV.130 and points out that readers are clearly to place Merteuil in the category of the "depraved" women Rosemonde criticizes.[42]

The physiological status of Valmont's aunt is important to our reading of this letter and to her categorization of female "depravity." Rosemonde is 80 years old and has thus gone "beyond womanhood." She is "immune" to passion, according to both her own estimation and the section "On Old Age and Death" of Laclos's essay "On Women." Just as important, she is to be understood as possessing an excellent mind, for we are told that she does by no less a judge of *esprit* than Merteuil, who chastises Valmont at one point in the novel for dismissing his aunt as "harsh and severe." Merteuil knows her old society ladies, she tells the Vicomte, for she is forced to spend time with them in order to establish her credentials as a full-fledged "prude." She declares Rosemonde to be one of those "rare and precious" old women with whom she willingly converses, for they have not neglected to "nourish their reason" and have thus created an existence for themselves "when nature's existence is missing." They possess "wise judgment, and a mind that is at one and the same time solid, gay, and gracious," along with a certain indulgence for human weakness born of their own youthful transgressions (261).

Rosemonde's indulgent, understanding, and above all well-reasoned letter is written to Tourvel just after the Présidente first has sex with Valmont, but as its placement indicates, her remarks on love are to be applied by the reader as much to Merteuil's as to Tourvel's situation. Men, Rosemonde writes, experience supreme pleasure in their own happiness, while women are made most happy by the pleasure they give to their partners. This difference, "so essential and so often ignored," is felt in the entirety of their relations but above all in the area of fidelity to the loved one: "The exclusivity of taste that characterizes love above all, is in men only a preference, serving at most to increase their pleasure, that with a different object would be lesser, but would not disappear." In women, the depth of feeling for the loved object makes all others repugnant, even those who should by rights engender desire. Rosemonde accordingly declares fidelity in women to be "stronger than nature, and removed from its empire" (304).

How exactly we are to understand "nature's empire" in this context is not clear. In "On Women," the "love" both sexes are said to experience in the state of nature ends when their physical needs are satisfied. Women as well as men move on

---

[41] Diaconoff presents Merteuil as in love and as consciously regretting her lost exclusivity with Valmont (*Eros and Power*, 43). Catherine Cusset, to the contrary, presents Merteuil as incapable of love: "Madame de Merteuil *knows* intellectually but cannot *experience* this kind of love" ("Editor's Preface," 5).

[42] Laclos, "Correspondance entre Madame Riccoboni et M. de Laclos," in *Oeuvres complètes*, 758.

to their next encounter with no second thoughts for the fleeting object of their previous "love." This same natural urge to have sex with all suitable male partners is apparently present in Rosemonde's women but is repressed when they are in love, or rather, turned into its opposite, repugnance. Thus the fidelity demonstrated by civilized women breaks with the omnipotence normally granted the state of nature, making love a powerful force indeed. This force is also to be understood, however, as somehow an inherent sexed difference, rather than a learned behavior. Rosemonde points as evidence to society's unspoken rule that men are excused for having sex with other partners, while women are condemned for doing the same. Men can be "unfaithful" without being "unconstant," a truism that Valmont of course incarnates, just as Tourvel incarnates faithful female love. In sum, for Rosemonde, the womanly ability to transcend natural lust is a rarefying, ennobling feature that speaks to the very "nature" of the female sex.[43] Those few women who have adopted male sexual comportment as their own—who are capable of loving one man while having sex with others—are, in Rosemonde's estimation, quite thoroughly depraved (*dépravées*, 304).

Even Cécile seems finally to realize this "truth" and to accept that Danceny will never be willing to marry her, however much he may "love" her, as illustrated by her decision to condemn herself to a cloistered life of repentance. Cécile's principal tormentor refuses to acknowledge the "natural" basis behind women's fidelity to men, however, or as she would put it, their capacity to confuse love with their lover. The monstrousness of Merteuil's character has often been attributed to her overly "masculine" traits: hard intelligence, aggressive sexuality, desire for mastery. Thomas Kavanagh has argued, to the contrary, that Merteuil should be viewed as highly feminine, an example, one might say, of Laclos's civilized woman *par excellence*, in that she is able to make men fall in love with her by pretending to be that which she is most decidedly not: as morally spotless on the inside as she is beautiful on the outside.[44] But Laclos also advises women to mirror internally the exterior qualities they exhibit, or pay the price for this disguise by losing the man they would fix to themselves. Nor does Merteuil need a "protector," it goes without saying; she is more than capable of protecting herself, as the Prévan episode famously illustrates (letter II.81 begins with her account of how she caused this legendary roué to be imprisoned). Her attempts to make men fall in love with her are aimed at controlling them while experiencing physical pleasure, making her a quite thoroughly twisted example of eighteenth-century womanhood according to both Mme de Rosemonde's intelligent assessment and the vision of civilized women presented in Laclos's essay.

---

[43]   The question of whether we are to accept that Valmont loves Tourvel has been much debated. Diaconoff, for example, sees Valmont as too narcissistic to be capable of love; she denies him the emotional evolution others have noted, writing that in the end he "seeks only what he had sought in the beginning: fame and glory and personal satisfaction" (*Eros and Power*, 49).

[44]   Kavanagh, "Educating Women," 150, 153.

Merteuil is *dépravée* in the sense of the dictionaries of the day: "spoiled," or "corrupt," a state literalized in the novel as an apparently latent, quite virulent case of smallpox. As Laclos states will always the case, Merteuil's exterior come to reflect her quite rotten interior, and the exposure is as dramatic as the deception was extreme. The idea that smallpox might be contained in a latent state in the body from birth was explored in the previous chapter, with regard to Julie's illness, and it is no surprise that like so many other eighteenth-century novelists, Laclos chose to use this powerful physical metaphor. Corruption and the body politic go hand in hand in Merteuil's case, for her latent illness may even be read as a sign of racial degradation, with the French nobility understood as a separate, doomed "race." Elizabeth Williams writes of Ménuret's work on inoculation against smallpox: "Enthusiastically embracing Bordeu's suggestion that smallpox was a seed that could germinate only in a given terrain, Ménuret posited the existence of a 'race' of smallpox sufferers—children born with a certain 'disposition of the organs, or constitution of the humors'—that made them prey to this affliction, just as there was a 'race of *Macrocéphales*' found in exotic lands."[45]

That Julie and Merteuil share this physical metaphor reveals its multivalence. Like Julie, Merteuil develops the illness from no discernible exterior source, but rather from an unbearable situation that brings to life a previously inert germ. The emotional catalyst for Merteuil involves being both booed at the theater (and thus effectively expelled from society) and losing an important judicial battle against her dead husband's heirs. But while Julie is spared any but the slightest scars, revealing that her guilt was unfounded, the damage to Merteuil is hideous to behold, a disfiguration perhaps meant to signify that she does indeed belong to a different "race" within the species of the human. There is a medical explanation for the unusual extent of her disfigurement, for we are told in a letter from Volanges to Rosemonde that the Marquise had contracted "confluent smallpox," a variety that causes the pustules to touch and join together in a matter of hours, to the extent that the entire body seems covered by one giant sore.

David Shuttleton notes that while discrete smallpox killed 25 percent of its victims, confluent smallpox carried away 75 percent of sufferers.[46] Of the few survivors, the majority were horribly disfigured. Pierre Darmon's striking description of the possible consequences includes Merteuil's loss of an eye:

> And what can one say of the scars that destroy the last vestiges of beauty: here, one sees the scalp falling off in strips, taking with it large quantities of hair; there, a one-eyed, pock-marked woman, or individuals with twisted limbs,

[45] Elizabeth A. Williams, *A Cultural History of Medical Vitalism in Enlightenment Montpellier* (Aldershot, UK and Burlington, VT: Ashgate, 2003), 225. The reference is to Ménuret de Chambord's *Advice for Mothers on Smallpox and Measles* (1769).

[46] See David Shuttleton, *Smallpox and the Literary Imagination, 1660–1820* (Cambridge: Cambridge University Press, 2007), 5.

cripples, and one-legged people whom a gangrenous smallpox has mutilated, offering at every moment the spectacle of illness and its consequences.[47]

The mention of "consequences" brings to mind the slippage noted by both Darmon and Shuttleton concerning the moral perfidy associated with syphilis (*la grande vérole*) and its "innocent" linguistic companion, *la petite vérole*. Darmon recounts the *bon mot* making the rounds when Louis XV was dying of smallpox—"There is nothing small among the great"—then makes the link to Merteuil: "In *les Liaisons dangereuses*, do not the lightning bolts of an avenging God strike the marquise de Merteuil by means of the ravages of the 'little sister'?"[48]

This reading is certainly to the point, but to view Merteuil's smallpox solely as a function of her sexual licentiousness is I believe to miss the central perversity of her character as a "civilized" woman. That we are meant to view her physical transformation as mirroring her exposure as a moral monster is indicated in the novel's final letter, in which Mme de Volanges cites a sharp-tongued marquis as having said of the disfigured social outcast: "Her soul is now on her face." Volanges adds: "Sadly, everyone found that the expression was fitting" (383). We might say that Merteuil has finally undergone the physical transformation that is said to accompany puberty: her essential, permanent temperament has been imprinted on her body in a clearly readable manner. She is no longer an illegible danger to her society.[49]

As for Tourvel's fate, her death may testify to her moral superiority, but it also reveals the damage that a highly degenerate culture can wreak upon those who incarnate moral worthiness, as Laclos would apparently have all French women attempt to do. Laclos's subsequent embrace of the Revolution and its values may reflect a more optimistic vision of the future for both men and women, for the best possible fate for the type of woman Laclos purports to address in "On Women and Their Education" is surely to be married to an equally virtuous man. This sort of man is described in an essay by another writer who would become active in Revolutionary events, Jean-Nicolas Démeunier, author of the *Spirit of the Usages and Customs of Different Peoples* (1776). Démeunier was elected to the 1789 Estates General and became active in Parisian Revolutionary politics before fleeing the Terror in 1792. He returned to France after the fall of Robespierre and was an important participant in the politics of the Consulate as well as the Napoleonic Empire. Démeunier's goal in this work is to demonstrate how so-called "polite" customs are merely the degenerate or "denaturalized" form of the usages of originary peoples. His title is an obvious homage to Montesquieu but he echoes Rousseau as well, as when he declares that love does not exist

---

[47]   Pierre Darmon, *La longue traque de la variole* (Paris: Perrin, 1987), 40.

[48]   Darmon, *La longue traque de la variole*, 54.

[49]   Many different readings of this conclusion exist; see for example Suellen Diaconoff, for whom the novel is a condemnation not only of this particular society but of human nature as a whole (*Eros and Power*, 2).

in the state of nature, but is rather the result of the heightening of the passions caused by the civilized lifestyle. For Démeunier, chastity and monogamy are the necessary social brakes on the lascivity that these heightened passions inspire. The evolution of the passions also leads, Démeunier insists, to the increasingly better treatment of women, for reasons centered on the needs of men: "As man becomes more civilized and his knowledge progresses, he is more sensitive to unhappiness and disappointment, he has a greater need for consolation; he appreciates companionship more, and one might say that the most enlightened and moral of peoples know best how to love" (81).

The vitalists and their peers, whether philosophers, physiologists, or both, were as concerned with the moral status of French men as they were with that of French women, however much women might function in the treatises and novels I have been examining—Merteuil among them—as so many indicators that French society had reached an untenable "end point" of civilization. The full blossoming of the "new woman" of the physiological texts relied on the simultaneous appearance of a new type of male partner, one perfectly suited to protecting and cherishing his relatively soft-bodied, soft-headed wife. As many historians have explored, the creation of such a "brave new world" began to seem somehow a real possibility as the century drew to a close and the monarchy began to crumble. The Revolution was, famously, as much an attempt to restart history, to begin again with the "Year One," as it was a political remaking of French society. The philosophy behind this masculine rebirth was quite similar to Laclos's advice to women in his essay: republican men were to "find themselves again" by listening to the dictates of natural law. In the following chapter, I explore the fate of one exceptional and exceptionally well-read woman, Marie-Jeanne Roland, as she attempted to negotiate the minefield of Revolutionary gender politics.

Chapter 5
Marie-Jeanne Roland, or Sexuality and the Republic of Virtue

> On the first day of May, when I was fourteen, nature bloomed suddenly, with no effort, like a lively fresh rose that opens to the first powerful rays of the springtime sun.
>
> —Marie-Jeanne Roland, *Private Memoir*

Marie-Jeanne Roland is considered the first French woman autobiographer in the modern sense, a distinction earned by the unusual openness to intimate revelation she exhibits in her *Private Memoir* (1795). Although she begins the work by denying that she is writing for publication, Roland knew that it would find an audience.[1] The circumstances in which she was writing—in the prisons of the Terror—ensured an interested, if not sympathetic audience. Her notoriety was a selling point as well, for Roland's arrest is in many ways attributable to a negative press campaign by journalists such Jean-Paul Marat, whose attacks against Roland were both heavily sexed and heavily sexual. In addition to portraying her as an interfering woman who had botched relations between the major political parties, Marat and others claimed that she was a harlot and accused her of sleeping with her husband's Girondin associates.

This husband was Jean-Marie Roland, who twice served as Minister of the Interior and twice resigned from this post. He was appointed first by Louis XVI, resigning in protest of the king's refusal to adhere to the goals of a constitutional monarchy. Following the king's arrest, Jean-Marie was reappointed to the post but resigned a second time in protest of the king's execution. The extent of his wife's involvement in Girondin activities is unclear, although she does admit in the *Private Memoir* to having written her husband's famous letter of resignation to the king and a number of other Girondin documents.[2] She insists however that because she allowed men to take public credit for her writings, she was innocent of the charge of improper meddling in affairs of state by a woman. Fully expecting to be released from prison, Marie-Jeanne Roland was instead found

---

[1]   The *Mémoires particuliers* is usually published with Roland's other prison writings, such as her "portraits" of Revolutionary political figures. Louis Bosc published the first, expurgated version of the *Mémoires particuliers* in 1795, under the title *Appel à l'impartiale postérité*. Claude Perroud produced a definitive critical edition in 1905, relied on by Paul de Roux, the editor of the far more accessible 1986 edition from which I am quoting.

[2]   For a detailed consideration of Roland's involvement in Revolutionary activities, see Chapter 3 of Susan Dalton's *Engendering the Republic of Letters* (Montreal: McGill-Queen's University Press, 2003).

guilty and her *Private Memoir* left unfinished when its author was guillotined on November 8, 1793.

In this chapter, I argue that the *Private Memoir* is "modern" not only for Roland's openness to intimate revelation but also for her skillful negotiation of the gender politics at play in the "two-sex" model of sexual differentiation. Above all, Roland's autobiography constitutes a tour-de-force effort to dissolve the contradictions inherent in a "new woman's" efforts to participate in the intellectual public sphere of her day. Roland is the ideal subject for this last chapter of my study for a number of reasons, including the prolific amount of writing she produced during her relatively short life. Her numerous published letters, essays, juvenilia, and other documents make her, in the words of Dorinda Outram, "probably the most extensively intimately documented woman of the French eighteenth century."[3] Most importantly in the context of my study, these writings reveal that Roland was well versed in the physiological theories of her day. She was particularly interested in childhood hygiene, even before she began to devote herself to raising her only child, daughter Eudora, 12 years old when her mother was executed.

As Marie-France Morel has noted, Roland had the knowledge and the confidence to debate medical matters with the doctors she knew and her letters often demonstrate her pride in having prevailed over their opinions. Morel even speculates that Roland could have become a doctor, given the amount of medical knowledge she possessed, had this professional avenue been open to her.[4] The *Private Memoir* is, understandably, a defense of the author's sexual and moral virtue, and I demonstrate in the first part of this chapter that Roland's self-defensive claims are based on the theories contained in the hygiene treatises I have been exploring. The vitalist physiology underlying her autobiographical self-portrait is most evident in the pages of the *Private Memoir* devoted to Roland's first menstrual period at age 14, described in the epigraph above as the sudden, effortless blooming of a rose. But while she insists repeatedly on her innate and highly exceptional femininity, Roland also includes "shocking" revelations explicitly modeled on the sexual disclosures found in the first six books of Jean-Jacques Rousseau's *Confessions* (1782). The most dramatic of these passages is an account of a young man who showed her his penis when she only 11, and later masturbated to orgasm by pressing against her.

Roland presents these episodes as having ensured her sexual virtue, encoded as complete ignorance, until her wedding night. As this twist on the standard eighteenth-century narrative of adolescent female development illustrates,

---

3   Dorinda Outram, *The Body and the French Revolution: Sex, Class and Political Culture* (New Haven: Yale University Press, 1989), 129. Future references in the text. For the standard biography, see Gita May, *Madame Roland and the Age of Revolution* (New York: Columbia University Press, 1970).

4   Marie-France Morel, "Mme Roland, sa fille, et les médecins: prime éducation et médicalisation à l'époque des lumières," *Annales de Bretagne* 86 (1979), 218.

Roland's account of her physico-moral character brings a unique perspective to bear on the "new woman" I have been exploring in this study. The manner in which Roland narrates her own life, her own moral development, her own physico-moral interconnectedness, reminds us that women were aware of and indeed were participating in the debate over the evolving meaning of sexual differentiation during this key moment in the history of ideas. Men more or less fully dominated the medical discourse on women during this period, and much of the literary discourse as well. Roland's incursions into these arguments, on the medical, literary, and political fronts make her a unique and fascinating subject for any study of late eighteenth-century womanhood. Roland was of course not the only woman actively negotiating Revolution gender politics, and I briefly consider another such public figure, Charlotte Corday, in the closing pages of this chapter. Roland was however the only woman to address her personal situation as a woman intellectual in such an informed manner and with such literary skill.

The Art of Resisting Enlightenment

Like Rousseau and many other intellectuals of the period, Roland tells her readers that Plutarch had been a revelation to her as a child: "At this moment were born the ideas and impressions that made me into a republican without my imagining that I was becoming one."[5] As this anachronistic model reveals (as much for her male counterparts as for herself), Roland never intended to present herself as embodying the "average" French woman of her day. Her famous declamation, supposedly addressed to an allegorical statue at the foot of the guillotine—"Oh Liberty! What crimes are committed in thy name!"—would seem, in the light of her *Private Memoir*, to apply above all to the waste of the talents of the one exceptional woman who would, moments later, mount the scaffold.

The editor of an early edition of this work clearly seizes the relationship between Roland's innate constitution and her moral exceptionality: "The most unpardonable crime committed during the Terror was, without contradiction, the murder of the Citizeness Roland; I am speaking less of the iniquity of the act than of the loss it represents to France ... She was given the most excellent dispositions by nature, she had so carefully cultivated them, that at eighteen she was already writing profoundly meditated reflections on abstract matters."[6] In the first part of her *Private Memoir*, Roland works to convince the reader that "nature" had indeed bestowed the ideal innate temperament upon her and that this gift had been carefully cultivated during her childhood and adolescence. As a result, we are

---

[5]   Marie-Jeanne Roland, *Mémoires particuliers*, in *Mémoires de Mme Roland* (Paris: Mercure de France, 1986), 313. Future references in the text. For a study of the early political leanings of Roland, see Kathryn Ann Kadane, "The Real Difference between Manon Phlipon and Madame Roland," *French Historical Studies* 3.4 (1963–1964), 542–9.

[6]   *Oeuvres de J. M. Ph. Roland*, ed. L. A. Champagneux, 3 vols (Paris: Bidault, 1800), I:i–ii.

invited to believe, she grew into a womanhood characterized by an unshakeable virtue combined with profound intellectual activity.

A brief biographical sketch of Roland's life is necessary here to provide a frame for her self-presentation in the *Private Memoir*. She was born Marie-Jeanne Phlipon in Paris in 1754 and enjoyed a comfortable bourgeois existence as the only child of a skilled engraver and a devoted mother. Her parents provided her with an excellent education, employing a number of private tutors. At the age of 25, she married the older and highly intellectual Jean-Marie Roland, an inspector of manufacturers. The couple often worked together, collaborating for example on Jean-Marie's magnum opus the *Dictionary of Manufacturers*, part of Charles-Joseph Panckoucke's *Methodical Encyclopedia by Order of Subject Matter* (a revision of Diderot and d'Alembert's *Encyclopédie*). In her *Private Memoir*, Roland describes (somewhat resentfully) working long hours on articles that would be attributed solely to her husband, just as she would continue to write for him when he became active in Revolutionary affairs.

After devoting herself for some time to her daughter, Roland became active in the events of the Revolution through her husband. On 1 June 1793, the National Assembly ordered the arrest of the Girondin delegates, a somewhat loose confederation, for various "crimes against the Republic." While her husband and his fellow Girdonins fled Paris, Roland chose to stay, a decision based on the mistaken belief that she faced no real danger. In the initial period of her incarceration, while Roland was still convinced that no harm would come to her and that she would soon be set free, she began work on a number of projects, including political sketches and musings on the course of the Revolution, and, of course, her *Private Memoir*. She at first claims in the *Private Memoir* to be writing "merely to pass the time," but when her impending execution causes her to breaks her story off abruptly just after her marriage, she writes: "Thirteen years spent in many different places, working continually, in contact with a great variety of individuals, and in the last years so close to the events of the day, would furnish the fourth and most interesting part of my memoir" (338).

Roland's account of her childhood, as I read it, is primarily designed to establish the intensity of her womanly virtue in what would have been the "most interesting" part of the *Private Memoir*. Of her parents' seven children, she writes, she was the second to be born and the only survivor. In establishing her exemplary health as a child, Roland begins very much in the beginning: *in utero*. At a time when pregnancy and childbirth were as dangerous for the mother as for the child, this fetus, we are told, was uniquely beneficial to her mother's physical condition: "My mother would often say complacently that I was the only one who never gave her any pain, for my delivery was as happy as her pregnancy: it seemed that I had improved her health" (204). Baby Marie-Jeanne was sent to a wet-nurse in the country, a woman chosen carefully for her "health and good morals," for immorality might be, it was believed, transmitted through breast milk. Lelland Rather cites a lecture by the Leiden physician Jerome Gaub (1747) on this topic: "Nor shall I recall how often the mind of a wellborn infant is corrupted by the milk of an immoral wet-nurse and inclined toward vices of the worst kind, completely foreign to its family stock."[7]

As a disciple of Rousseau, Roland would of course keep baby Eudora at home and breastfeed her, but she stresses that the country setting of her own infancy contributed to her overall health. Brought back to Paris after two years of rustic living, she tells us, she had to be taught how to use a chamber pot, having been accustomed to retiring to a corner in the yard. The contrast between the country and the city established by this anecdote is a common theme in the *Private Memoir*; Roland is simultaneously proud of the sophistication that her Parisian upbringing gave her, and of her ability to adapt with ease to a simpler existence, including provincial life on her husband's country estate, Le Clos de la Platière.

We are next treated to a portrait-in-words of the young Mlle Phlipon, or "Manon," as her parents called her. Roland paints this portrait after explaining that she will not do so, as it must be of no interest to the reader: "One would not expect me to paint a portrait at this point of a little brunette girl of two, whose black hair contrasted so well with the high color of her lively face, and who embodied the happiness of her age, of which she enjoyed all the health. I know a better time to give my portrait and I am not so maladroit as to do so prematurely" (204–5). Temperament was not fixed in a child, for it required the tumultuous revolution of puberty to settle an individual's adult physiology, and Roland goes on to offer a lengthier postpuberty portrait later in the work; but neither was she so "maladroit" as to miss the opportunity to note the "high color" exhibited by her toddler self, that of the healthy, sanguine child described in the physiological treatises of the day. The young Manon is indeed the very picture of childhood sanguinity, and as Daignan notes, should such a child be protected from the ravages of "climate, food, education, and accidents … that change the fundamentals of their primitive constitution," she will become "truly sanguine" as an adult.[8]

Roland was interested in medicine for practical as well as theoretical purposes, for she tended to the medical needs of the families on her husband's estate. Although the common practice was to send one's sick tenant farmers to the (questionable) charity of the *hôpital*, at Le Clos de la Platière the mistress of the house served as doctor. Françoise Kermina comments: "She kept up her charitable works at all stages of her life. At Le Clos, she herself cared for her farmers instead of sending them to the hospital as was commonly done. 'My wife is the apothecary of the canton,' Roland would say, who found her overly generous."[9] The birth of her daughter precipitated a more intense investigation into infant and childhood hygiene. She sought out as much information on the proper method of raising

---

[7]   Lelland Rather, *Mind and Body in Eighteenth-Century Medicine: A Study Based on Jerome Gaub's* De regimine mentis (Berkeley: University of California Press, 1965), 102.

[8]   Guillaume Daignan, *Tableau des variétés de la vie humaine*, 2 vols (Paris: chez l'Auteur, 1786), 99.

[9]   Françoise Kermina, *Madame Roland ou la passion révolutionnaire* (Evreux: Librarie Académique Perrin, 1976), 92.

children as she could find, writing at one point to ask Louis Bosc his opinion of Arnaud Berquin's moral tales in *The Children's Friend* (1782–1783), which she knew only from reading reviews.[10] She also mentions reading and rereading the *Emile* and the *Encyclopédie*, as well as consulting Marie-Angélique Anel Le Rebour's *Advice for Mothers Wishing to Nurse Their Children* (1767) after her milk ran dry.[11] Le Rebours was a midwife and a mother herself, and her popular work in favor of the health benefits of nursing went through a number of editions by 1800.

Roland was even personally acquainted with one of the most famous authors of a work on childhood hygiene, Jacques Ballexserd. A Genevan watchmaker as well as a physiologist, Ballexserd was a friend of Roland's father, Gatien Phlipon, an engraver of some talent. Ballexserd was a frequent visitor to the Phlipon household, and attempted to convince Roland's parents to have their daughter inoculated against smallpox. He failed in his efforts and, as a result, she contracted the dreaded disease at the age of 16. That she came through this experience with only mild discomfort is yet another proof offered to the reader of her outstanding physical health. The numerous specialized medical terms she includes in the description of her bout with smallpox are perhaps intended as well to demonstrate the adult autobiographer's medical knowledge:

> They feared that I would develop complications from putrid fever and small pox. I had miliary fever and, the eruption peculiar to this type working against the other eruption, the smallpox gave me only a few large sores that flattened out without any pus and left only dry scabs that fell off easily. Doctor *Missa* told me that the Italians call this type of smallpox *ravaglioni*, or false pus-producing sores; they left no traces on me; and in fact the polish of my skin was not even altered by this illness, although this noxious humor, after the danger was past, caused a state of languor that remained for four or five months. (272)

Each time an illness arises in those around her, as in the case of her mother's premature death (attributed by Roland in part to the stresses of menopause), the reader of the *Private Memoir* is treated to a succinct medical diagnosis, one that often contradicts that of the attending physician. Roland attributes the death of one of her tutors, for example, to his doctor's unwise prescription of bloodletting at an inappropriate moment: "A bleeding given at the wrong season caused the gout from which he suffered to settle in his chest, killing him at the age of fifty" (208).

The space allocated to Roland's account of her passage through the "revolution" of puberty illustrates her knowledge of the hygiene treatises as well, for this event is presented as the most significant physical experience of her early years. We are

---

[10]   Arnaud Berquin's 12 volumes of moralizing tales considered fit for children were immensely popular in both France and England up through the nineteenth century (*L'Ami des enfants*, 12 vols [London: Elmsley, 1782–1783]).

[11]   Letter of 19 January 1785, in *Lettres de Madame Roland*, ed. Claude Perroud, 2 vols (Paris: Imprimerie Nationale, 1900–1902), I:485.

not surprised to find that the details of her account concur with the best possible scenario outlined in the period's many treatises on the subject. Roland approaches her story by noting the increasing development of her intellectual faculties at this stage of her development, although she has been stressing her intellectual precociousness all along (she tells us that she learned to read "before the age of four" and was from then on essentially an autodidact, although tutors were brought in to instruct her in a few disciplines):

> The development of my intellect was accompanied by natural developments of other kinds. On the first day of May, when I was fourteen, nature bloomed suddenly, with no effort, like a lively fresh rose that opens to the first powerful rays of the springtime sun ... I noticed it with a kind of joy, as if I were entering the class of grownups, and I announced it to my mother who embraced me tenderly, thrilled to see me traverse so brilliantly a passage that had worried her for my health. (251)

While far more subtle and even poetic than the physiological texts to which it refers, this passage has a clear message to send to the informed reader. In order to experience so few symptoms at puberty, Roland would have had to possess a purity of mind recommended by all the physiological writers of the day, but achieved, as they all stress, by few city-dwelling young girls. How, in her Paris setting, with access to the works of the most progressive authors of her day— she informs us that her mother made no attempt to censure her reading, other than keeping *The New Heloise* from her, fearing that it would have too strong an emotional effect—did Manon pull off this remarkable feat?

The explanation is to be found in the least likely of the childhood experiences that Roland recounts: an incident of sexual abuse that took place in her tenth year. Roland prefaces this passage in a manner that leaves no doubt as to its importance. She has just begun to discuss her increasing interest in religion at this period in her life, but interrupts herself as follows: "A circumstance too important to my moral development for me to skip over it came to add to my anxieties and inspire in me a great resolution" (217). She tells us that a 16-year-old apprentice in her father's workshop had, when the two were momentarily (and unusually) alone, forced her hand to touch an "extraordinary thing" under a workbench. He had then shown this "thing" to her. When she became upset, he told her that she was overreacting. In a later conversation, he informed her that "your mother plays that way with your father, and is not afraid," to which she responded: "That's not true, that's too naughty. —I swear to you that I am certain of it, but they do it differently; I'll tell you how, if you want. —I don't want to know, leave me alone" (218).

This was merely the first incident of two, however, and the second had a far greater impact on the young girl's psyche:

> One day, when my father had made me work for a few minutes with him and had then been suddenly called outside, I was about to leave the workshop after him when some sort of fanfare sounded from the Pont-Neuf quite close to where

we lived. I stepped up onto a stool by the window because I could not see properly. 'Climb onto the edge of the bench,' said the young man, helping me to do so. The others went out to see what was happening. He stood behind me and when I started to get down he put his hands under my arms and lifted me up, pressing me against himself in such a way that my skirts were pushed up and I found myself sitting on his knees, as he himself sat back on a chair at the same moment. I then felt this extraordinary thing behind me. 'Let me go, sir,' I cried. 'What?' he said, 'Are you still afraid? I'm not doing you any harm.' 'But I want to go. My dress —.' 'Never mind your dress, I'll see to that.' He then put his hand where nothing else had been and started to caress me. I struggled, trying to push his arms away and change my position, and managed to slip my feet to the ground. Then I caught sight of his face. I was horrified. His eyes were starting from his head and he was breathing hard. I nearly fainted. He noticed my emotion, and his crisis probably over, he assumed a gentle air and tried his best to calm me, not wanting me to leave until he had done so. He finally did; but instead of increasing my curiosity in this way, the liberties he had taken excited my repugnance. (219)

In comparison to the paradigms of female seduction discussed in the previous chapters, whereby a young girl's encounter with lascivious behavior triggers an immediate awakening of sexual desire and the curiosity to explore these feelings, every detail of this passage points to Manon's lack of response, as well as to her lack of culpability. She had been about to follow her father out of the workshop, but had been held back by an eminently childlike curiosity in a noisy street scene of some sort. She apparently did not know that the other apprentices had gone out with her father, for she had been looking out of the window. Add to these circumstances the rapidity of the young man's attack, the immediacy of her demands to be released, and above all her now extinct intellectual curiosity as to what her parents did when alone, and we are witnessing a perfectly excusable scene of an unwanted encounter with a young man's "extraordinary thing."

Roland's treatment of this episode seems exceedingly modern in some aspects, as when she goes on to explore how this event affected her young psyche. She tells us that her previous penchant for religious excess now blossomed into a demand to be sent to a convent school for instruction, the better to prepare herself for her first communion. That was what she told her parents, and what she believed; her true motive, however, understood only in retrospect, was to escape a world containing men: "I fell into a devotion that changed me in strange ways; I was profoundly humble, inexpressibly timid; I looked upon men with a sort of terror that increased when they seemed pleasing to me; I watched over my thoughts with excessive scrupulousness" (220). This scrupulousness survived into her teenage years, we are told, despite her (brief) period as an atheist. So eager was she to avoid all further information concerning the employ of that "extraordinary thing," she tells us, that at age 16 she flipped past the plates of Buffon's *Natural History* devoted to anatomy with a speed inspired by terror (she does not mention avoiding the section of this enormous treatise devoted to puberty, including those concerning the physiology of girls and women).

Capping these ramifications of the apprentice's behavior, Roland makes an astonishing statement concerning the shock that awaited her on her wedding night: "I finally married at the age of twenty-five, and with a soul such as one might assume, highly inflammable senses, and much instruction in many areas, I had so well avoided increasing my knowledge of the one area in which I had begun so prematurely, that the events of the first night of my marriage were as surprising to me as they were disagreeable" (221). She stresses later in the *Private Memoir* that she was not completely ignorant; she of course knew where babies came from, just not the precise details as to how they got there: "I was fond of reading the Bible, and I often went back to it: our old translations often express things as crudely as do doctors … This put me on the path of a type of instruction that is rarely given to young girls; but it was presented in a manner that had nothing seductive to it, and I had too much to think about to concentrate on a purely material matter that seemed disagreeable to me" (211–12). As for the marriage night, she knew enough to expect to feel pleasure (the source of this knowledge is not specified), but was disappointed not only in this expectation, but in her nascent stoicism as well: "My wedding night overturned all my pretensions, preserved until that moment; although surprise played a role in all this; a novice stoic would not need to be as strong when facing suffering she had expected, as in facing pain that struck suddenly when she had been expecting quite the contrary" (256).

Roland is not telling us of the consequences of this abuse in order to convince us that she was psychically damaged—far from it. She is certainly inviting our sympathy for her younger self, and is quite adamant as to how difficult it is to recount the story—she claims that it is far harder for her than was Rousseau's most painful revelation in his *Confessions*—but her main goal is to convince the reader that this episode guaranteed her absolute innocence of the mechanics of intercourse until her wedding night. In a lovely, paradoxical move, the workshop incident is the proof of Roland's highly desirable innocence. She stresses elsewhere how entirely she was protected from Parisian decadence, telling us that she never left the house unchaperoned as a single woman, even after her mother died. She is in other words not arguing against the legitimacy of the belief that exposure to licentiousness is the key to moral and physical degeneration. She is arguing that her extreme shock and disgust at the workshop incident, coupled with a profound ignorance as to why she was shocked and disgusted, ensured her continuing virtue alongside the protection afforded her by her parents and her own natural inclinations. These inclinations included a youthful penchant for religious ecstasy, for she tells us that following the incident, "religious ideas dominated in me; the reign of sentiment, hastened by my already precocious leanings, took the form of the love of God, the sublime delirium of which beautified and preserved the first years of my adolescence, resigned the others years to philosophy, and seems to have thus protected me forever from the storms of passion" (220).

Yet another "shocking" revelation comes when Roland relates what amount to female "wet dreams" as she approaches prepuberty. She tells us that just before her first menstrual period, "I had on several occasions been drawn from a profound sleep in a surprising manner. Imagination played no part in this; I was exercising it upon too many serious things, and my timorous conscience was keeping it so carefully from other subjects, that it was impossible for me to imagine that which I had not allowed myself to try to understand" (251). Roland apparently did not mention these experiences to her mother, although she did turn to her confessor for information on this curious topic. He affirmed her belief that these incidents were sent by God to test her virtue, just as He had tested the tormented Saints in the desert, for whose trials she now had, she tells us, an increased sympathy.

Roland's tortured syntax ("it was impossible for me to imagine that which I had not allowed myself to try to understand") echoes her earlier account of sexual abuse and is similarly designed to indicate that her virtuous young mind instinctively resisted knowledge of a sexual nature. Her claim that "imagination" played no role in instigating these events is highly significant as well, for "imagination" is the closest equivalent in the eighteenth-century French lexicon to the Freudian unconscious. As Jean Starobinksi has written: "Despite what is fairly widely believed today, it was quite usual to speak of the unconscious before Freud's time, but it was an unconscious associated with the obscure murmurings of visceral functions, from which would emerge, intermittently, conscious acts."[12] "Imagination" is to be understood as the part of the mind most resistant to the control of reason, tending to shoot off in undesirable directions despite one's best efforts at self-control. As such, it is tightly linked to the senses, is indeed that part of the mind that is most in the thrall of bodily sensations.

In Laclos's *On Women*, he claims that his young girl in the state of nature completely lacks this mental faculty, held responsible for the degradation of eighteenth-century French girls in whom its fire "almost never fails to be set alight."[13] To prove the absence of "imagination" as a factor in her nighttime emissions, Roland tells us that when she was so "rudely" awakened by these sensations, it was from "a deep sleep"—no dreaming involved. She does admit that she did not at first put an immediate stop to these pleasurable sensations upon awakening, a lapse that caused her intense religious guilt. She soon trained herself, however, to awaken at the first stirring of pleasure, at which point she would jump out of bed, barefoot, and "in spite of the winter cold, with my arms in the form of a cross, I would pray to the Lord to preserve me from the traps of the demon" (252). The next day, she would put ashes in her bread as penance.

The 39-year-old autobiographer is amused by such youthful excesses. She explains that the horror felt by her devout 14-year-old self was quite misplaced, for these pleasurable feelings had been quite divorced from licentious thoughts. Using terms worthy of any eighteenth-century physiological treatise, Roland explains that these sensations were produced when "an extraordinary boiling roused my

---

[12]   Jean Starobinski, "A Short History of Bodily Sensation," in *Fragments for a History of the Human Body* (New York: Zone Books, 1989), III:364.

[13]   Choderlos de Laclos, "Des Femmes et de leur éducation," in *Oeuvres complètes* (Paris: Gallimard, 1979), 399.

senses during the heat of rest and, strengthened by my excellent constitution, operated a purification within me that was as unknown to me as its cause" (251). It was the purely physical heat generated by her sleeping young body, overheated under her blankets, which brought on these events, by "boiling" her oh-so-healthy adolescent blood. These emissions were merely physical discharges, and as such, highly desirable in a healthy young girl approaching puberty; so many healthy excretions working to purify her body of excremental excess as it reached the necessary state of plethora that would soon cause "nature to bloom."

That there was a "liquid" produced during these events is an important detail of Roland's account, for it is meant to indicate that she "ejaculated." As mentioned in Chapter 2, many eighteenth-century physiologists believed that women produced a semen-like substance at orgasm, although the much reduced quantity of this ejaculate in comparison to the male orgasm made it far less interesting as a physiological phenomenon. The theory that ejaculation not brought on by the "imagination" was a healthy phenomenon is found in Ménuret's *Encyclopédie* article "Manustupration": "masturbation that is not frequent, that is not excited by a boiling and voluptuous imagination, and is in the end the result of need, does not give rise to any problems and is not an Evil (for medicine)."[14] Roland is following this theory in that she clearly insists that the loss of genital fluid during these nighttime orgasms was a sign of her brilliant health, and certainly not caused by "manual stupration" or licentious dreams, for it was "impossible for her to imagine that which she had not allowed herself to try to understand."

The opportunity to dwell on such amusing memories, Roland goes on to tell her readers, makes her almost happy to be in prison, and able to divert herself with scenes she never otherwise would have had the time to recall. She then goes on to draw a verbal portrait of her young, devout, needlessly frightened, and needlessly guilty self, making of this combination a voluptuous image of sexualized innocence worthy of a novelist, or of a physiologist carried away in his description of the splendor of his ideal French virgin: "How humble and fervent I was, when *that* happened to me! How much my voice, my timid countenance, my yet more animated complexion, those humid shining eyes must have added to the expression of a physiognomy that breathed candor and sensibility! What a mix of innocence, premature feelings, good sense, and simplicity!" (252). She tells us, predictably, that even these (relatively) innocuous events worked to fortify her virtue. She became "mistress of her imagination" as a result of her efforts to anticipate and control these overwhelming physical experiences and soon developed a solid and lasting immunity to any "surprise" of the senses: "I view pleasure, like happiness, only in the union of that which charms both the heart and the senses and brings on no regrets ... but that does not shelter me from what they call a passion, and it may be that it even makes the passion more enduring. I could add

---

[14] "Manustupration," in *Encyclopédie, ou Dictionnaire raisonné des sciences, des arts et des métiers*, ed. Denis Diderot and Jean d'Alembert (Paris: Briasson [etc.], 1751–1765), X:51.

here, like the geometricians, 'that is what must be demonstrated' [*C. C. Q. F. D.*]. Patience! We have time to arrive at the proof' (253).

This exhortation to patience on the reader's part is a reference to Roland's famous and (probably) unconsummated passion for François Buzot, the Revolutionary leader who would kill himself a short time after her execution. Roland did not have "enough time to arrive at the proof," of course, enough time to treat the reader to an explanation of just how this virtue-fortified woman, immune to the pleasures of the senses but not to a "passion," fell desperately in love, only to remain faithful to an unappreciative husband. Part of the preparation for this "most interesting" material is her claim of developing superior willpower, for as she moves into the postpuberty period, Roland's treatment of her moral makeup begins to reach an adult complexity. Her self-portrayal becomes, that is, less physiologically bound and more psychologically rich. This shift also reflects the physiological writings of her day in that as a young person reached full growth and development, her personality, or temperament, was believed to solidify and stabilize, allowing her mind to take on a (relatively) independent life of its own.

There are hints of this strong, self-assured woman in Roland's account of her life up until the age of 25. Roland repeats many of the physiological commonplaces when describing her younger self, as when she refers to the "desire to please that lifts up the budding breast, that makes one feel a sweet sensation at the flattering looks one notices one is receiving," but she insists that her superior intellect acted to modify these general, inescapable feminine traits for the better. We are told that she made a "singular" impression on those who met her, for this natural desire to please, "combined with my timidity and my modesty and the austerity of my principles, spread over my person, and leant to my toilette a very particular charm" (255). But even as a young girl, she tells us, she was able to reflect on the nature of vanity and thus to combat its force, asking herself: "Is it thus to shine for others, like decorative flowers, and receive vain praise, that those of my sex are raised to virtue? — What does it mean, this extreme desire to please that devours me, and leaves me unhappy even when it should be satisfied? ... Ah! no doubt, I am destined for better things" (264).

While we are not to think that this young girl had any plans other than to become an ideal wife and mother, the older narrator is hardly content to present her younger self as "merely" a normal young girl, a healthy physico-moral "machine" conforming in every way to the physiologists' limited vision of women's intellectual powers. Men were said to be set apart from women by their ability to overcome their dependency on their bodies, or, to put the matter more precisely, the makeup of their bodies was said to grant their minds more independence of judgment. Men were accordingly presented as less subject to the extravagances of sensibility, and indeed to all internal "compulsions" as well as external forces such as climate.

Faced with this extreme moral and physical dichotomy, Roland would have it both ways: she claims to possess the moral and intellectual strengths clearly labeled "masculine" in her day, but reserves the right to remain entirely, even paradigmatically, a woman. The champions of women among the male philosophical elite of the eighteenth century rarely went so far as to grant women intellectual parity with men. Antoine-Léonard Thomas, for example, obviously viewed himself as a panegyrist of women's virtues, for his stated goal in the *Essay on the Character, Mores, and Mind of Women in Different Centuries* was to discover "to what qualities and various types of merit women are susceptible, to what heights government, circumstances, and laws may elevate them, and the secret relationship between politics and women's morals."[15] But while he frequented the salons of some of the most admired women intellectuals of his day, including those of Marie-Thérèse Geoffrin, Julie de Lespinasse, and Suzanne Necker, Thomas does not praise women's wit and intelligence in his essay. He reserves admiration for those contemporary women who do good works for the poor and for young married beauties who spend their time caring for their own children rather than seeking lovers. He declares: "Oh! If these examples could bring back nature and morals among us!" (85).

Thomas admits that only a few individuals can be counted as true geniuses, but emphasizes that these individuals have all been men. Women are said to have superior imaginations, but to be incapable of using this hypersensibility to create artistic works. The physiological cause Thomas gives for this incapacity is that cited by the physiologists: the natural weakness of their organs that causes them to be highly nervous and to receive a multitude of (distracting) sensations. While these weak organs also give rise to their soft beauty and attractive gaiety, their fluidity prevents "that strong and sustained attention capable of combining a long chain of ideas, that obscures all other objects in order to see only one in its entirety" (42). Thomas concludes that woman's imagination "reflects everything, and creates nothing" (45).

Embodying Republican Contradictions

Roland was aware of the contradiction inherent in her claim to possess intellectual superiority alongside all the (positive) traits labeled "feminine" by her culture. In her *Private Memoir*, she often foregrounds her practical efforts to negotiate this contradiction, without, of course, presenting these efforts as a part of a protofeminist agenda. The result is a vision of a woman who adheres to quite conservative standards of female behavior, while living a "secret" life of amazing intellectual daring. She exults in the contrast that her tasteful bourgeois attire and downcast eyes present to the hidden intellectual ferment of her mind, and nowhere more so than when she describes herself sitting demurely in church, hiding her Helvétius, Voltaire, Spinoza, Diderot, Descartes, or Malebranche in her missal.

As she pursued this extraordinary autodidactic program, she says, she adopted alternating systems of belief. She says of reading Helvétius: "He destroyed

---

[15] Antoine-Léonard Thomas, *Essai sur le caractère, les moeurs, et l'esprit des femmes dans les différents siècles* (Paris: Champion, 1987), 4. Future references in the text.

my most ravishing illusions; he made everything repugnantly interesting." She responded by persuading herself that he was painting "men as they had become through the corrupting influence of society" (256). Her period of true atheism, we are told, began sometime between the ages of 14 and 16 (in perfect timing with the full awakening of her intellectual capacities at puberty, we note). In later life, she became what is perhaps best described as a deist, for she writes that she is convinced that there is more to life than materialism can explain. Always, however, she followed the outward practices of the religion dictated by her cultural situation, attending Catholic services regularly, whether under her father's or her husband's dominion, and regardless of their own neglect of what she considered her civic responsibility.

The effort to place this philosophy of a double life within the context of gendered Revolutionary politics has dominated recent discussions of Roland's work, for she was clearly negotiating, in both her life and her writings, the rapidly changing rules of the "public sphere" of French cultural politics. The most important gender-focused treatment of Roland's *Private Memoir* from the perspective of my own concerns is the chapter devoted to this work in Dorinda Outram's *The Body in the French Revolution* (1989). Outram's study overall focuses on the "public embodiment" of the Revolutionaries, a process of representation she links to the Montpellier revolution in medicine. She sees the vitalists' rejection of Cartesian dualism as mirroring the republican rejection of the tenet that the French king was divinely appointed, and argues that in the absence of a transcendent "soul," the self-appointed leaders of the body politic needed to set themselves apart, and did so by emphasizing their stoic virtue. As willpower was, like intellect and reason, a virtue unavailable to the "new woman," it follows that whatever her political views, a woman interested in participating in Revolutionary events faced the problem of, as Outram puts it, "how to achieve effective public personification when the entire realm of public dignity had been defined in a specifically male way through the use of the male body-image" (85).

I part company with Outram when she diagnoses Roland as displaying an "efficient internalization of the idea that women can only have a public existence in as much as they wield corrupt power" (147). That the mistresses of the ancien régime kings had wielded corrupt power was a well-worn Revolutionary cliché, with which Roland would have been well acquainted, but I disagree that she was forced into a confused self-identification with women such as Madame de Pompadour. Nor do I agree that Roland viewed herself as stuck with "a difficult female body," one so lacking the autonomy of the male body that she felt "invaded" by her husband during sex, then by the child growing within her, and finally by the milk that she needed to produce to nourish her child in accordance with the latest standards of ideal motherhood.[16] Outram concludes that only in prison is Roland able to view herself as "an uncontroverted whole," a reading that, carried to its

---

[16]   On Roland's view of motherhood, see Lesley Walker "Sweet and Consoling Virtue: The Memoirs of Madame Roland," *Eighteenth-Century Studies* 34.3 (2001): 403–19.

conclusion, makes the fate of death by guillotine ultimately preferable to sex or breast-feeding: cleaner, more independent, and spectacularly public.[17]

While I very much agree with Outram's view of Roland as responding to her culture's view of feminine virtue, I argue that Roland's vision of her body was not subject to the fluctuations of the Revolutionary cultural imagination but rather fixed in the latest scientific findings and the most up-to-date philosophizings on the mind–body relationship. More importantly, I see her as actively transforming her culture's prescriptions concerning the female body to her own ends and doing so in a quite conscious manner. Take for example the workshop scene, the first physical experience narrated in the *Private Memoir*, as Outram points out. Outram interprets the scene as the young Roland having "partly encouraged, partly rejected, the fumbling physical contact offered her by one of her father's apprentices, intrigued, yet terrified that the young man would bring their meetings to their logical conclusion" (132). The long-term psychological consequence of this trauma for Outram is that Roland is left, even as she writes this passage at age 39, confused as to her chastity. Roland's attitude toward her role in Revolutionary politics is then diagnosed as similarly ambivalent: "Unable to define herself as either chaste or unchaste, Mme Roland's attitude to the influence she did wield during her husband's brief tenure of office was equally ambiguous" (133).

My own reading of this scene is obviously quite different. While Roland may have been "intrigued" by the first incident with the apprentice, her narrative communicates that what fascinates her younger self is the possibility that her parents engage in similar behavior, not that she may have the opportunity to do so in the future. This point is important, for the narrating Roland quite vehemently stresses her absolute ignorance of the use to which the young man might put his "extraordinary thing." We are certainly not obliged to take her at her word, but there is no textual evidence to the contrary. Roland is also careful to justify having found herself alone with the apprentice a second time by explaining that a passing "fanfare" had distracted her and that, following the rather violent groping that was then inflicted upon her (not "offered" to her), she refused even to dine with the other members of the household, instead eating alone with her mother. In the end, she begged to be sent to a convent school, where she would be securely protected from any further encounters with young men—although again, the older narrator insists that her younger self felt only a religious euphoria and was unaware that her request was motivated by a desire to avoid such "extraordinary things." She ends her account with a stirring call to mothers to consider the "frightening" extent of the vigilance required of them in watching over their daughters. The "ignorance or inclination, even the ingenuousness of the innocence" of these young creatures is said to expose them to "the audacious enterprises of a sex that is always brutal should a well-chosen education not inspire in it either severe morals or great delicacy" (222).

---

[17]   Roland's struggles to breastfeed her daughter are recounted in letters to her husband from 29 November 1781 until 16 January 1782, as well as in her essay *Avis à ma fille en âge et dans le cas de devenir mère*, written shortly after the birth of her daughter.

All of these details, including the maternal exhortation, are designed to argue for the continuing physical and more importantly moral chastity of Roland's younger self. The autobiographical narrator is intent on presenting the 11-year-old Manon as quite untouched by licentiousness. Roland indeed seems to take on this scene as a deliberate tour-de-force of confessional writing. She begins her account: "I am a bit embarrassed by what I am about to relate, for I want my work to be chaste, given that my person has never ceased to be so, and yet, what I must tell is not very chaste at all" (217). I read this statement not as a confused admission of unchastity but to the contrary as a quite Rousseauian signal to the reader that despite what Roland is about to relate, both her child self and her *Private Memoir* will indeed remain chaste.[18] Like Rousseau, she reveals "all," sparing herself nothing, and, like Rousseau, this "all" reveals only an exceptionally virtuous person triumphing over adversity. That this person was also a woman only added to Roland's challenges as an autobiographer, but she gladly took on such challenges, it would appear, and relished the *seeming* contradictions that she then explodes, just as Rousseau's *Confessions* lays bare his apparent transgressions only to argue that they are anything but evidence of personal corruption.

In arguing for her virtue, Roland was relying on yet another aspect of her culture's understanding of physiology: the possibility of exceptions to the rule. As a species, human beings were said to stand out among animals for their ability to "go beyond" nature. It is in their nature, so to speak, to do so, at least according to Roussel, as quoted in Chapter 2: "Reason and will detach man from the great chain that links all other beings; and the imperceptible strings that attach him to it still, are lax enough to permit him to distance himself a bit at times from the exact and straight path that the others are obligated to follow" (305). Roussel even presents exceptional individuals as freed by their "particular properties" from certain, unspecified "general laws" to which all others are subject: "The more bodies possess those particular properties that distinguish them from common matter, the more they appear to be independent of the general laws that guide it" (303).

It is highly doubtful that Roussel had women in mind when he wrote these phrases, or that in his view a woman who did not adhere to all of the "laws" of nature with regard to her sex would have been considered "exceptional" in the positive sense of that term. Thomas, as seen above, allowed women to excel only in the quality of their imagination, and would not for all that grant them superior creativity. Françoise Kermina seizes Roland's dilemma with great clarity: "It was necessary to acquire the qualities needed to serve society while understanding that one would never be able to use them ... to demonstrate as brilliantly as possible that women were not supposed to be brilliant" (51). As I have been arguing, Roland had a solution to this problem, and a consciously elaborated solution: she would indulge herself in intellectual pursuits only when the witnesses to her talents were close friends who could be trusted both to value her superiority and to hide it from others. In a letter to Bosc of 1785, for example, Roland admonishes him not to

---

[18]   Outram, *The Body and the French Revolution*, 133.

reveal her true position on religion. She describes how she deals with her devout brother-in-law, nodding and smiling while he rambles on about religious matters, gestures he takes to indicate agreement.[19]

Hypocrisy? To the contrary, as she explains in her *Private Memoir* when she describes her adoption of this philosophy of doubleness:

> In the midst of doubts, uncertainties, and research relative to these great questions, I quickly decided that the *unity* of the inner self, if I can call it so, that is, the greatest agreement between one's opinions and one's conduct, was a necessary part of an individual's wellbeing; one must thus examine what is right and, when decided on this question, practice it rigorously. Now, there is a kind of justice to be observed with oneself when one would live alone in the world; one should regulate one's personal feelings, so as to be the slave of no one. A being is *good* in itself, when all its parts are working together toward self-preservation, toward maintenance or improvement: that is true for the moral as well as the physical realms. Health consists of the proper arrangement of the parts, of the equilibrium of the humors; it is preserved by healthy food and moderate exercise. One's moral constitution is formed by the proportions of desire and the harmony of the passions, and only wisdom can ensure the excellence and continuation of a good moral balance. Its first principles are to be found in what most benefits the individual, and in this regard, one can truthfully say that virtue is only the application of reason to morality.
>
> But virtue properly understood is born only out of one's relationships with one's fellow beings; one is wise for oneself, virtuous with regard to others. In society, everything is relative, there is no longer independent happiness; one is required to sacrifice a part of the happiness one might otherwise enjoy to avoid risking the loss of all one's happiness and in order to preserve a portion of it from all attempts to destroy it. (258–9)

That Roland's central metaphor is medical gives the passage an objective tone, and places her relationship to public virtue very much in the context of hygiene theory. She is managing her "moral constitution" according to a vitalist model of the balance of internal humors with external influences. In the "microclimate" of her private life, she will be "the slave of no one," regulating her feelings with her own best interests in mind. Wisdom will be her goal and her intellect her chief guide. When in public, "virtue" becomes the all-powerful guide to her actions, understood according to society's view of this attribute in women, not according to her own private musings on the virtuous life. But while she thus "enslaves" herself by conforming to her society's dictates even when they contradict her carefully reasoned opinions, she does so in conformation with her philosophy of the public/ private divide. Most importantly, this public enslavement functions to preserve the precious happiness she feels when she can divorce herself from such concerns in her (equally virtuous) private existence.

---

[19]   Letter of 23 March 1785, in *Lettres*, I:507.

The situational irony of Roland's imprisonment while she writes this passage is hardly lost on the reader, or on the autobiographer herself. Something has gone terribly wrong with her plan to keep the "socially inappropriate" aspects of her private happiness out of the reach of those who would attack her for them. She ascribes this crisis to a betrayal: someone has handed over proof to the authorities that she was the true author of several crucial Girondin documents. In so doing they have committed a terrible injustice against her and forced her to justify herself when she would rather "be reading a chapter of Montaigne, drawing a flower, or playing an arietta, relieving the solitude of my prison existence without having to work at my confession" (305). That she had never had the slightest intention of letting the public know that she had written some of her husband's work makes all the difference, or should, according to the ethics outlined above. Now that she is in prison and has been publicly charged, she is forced to go "beyond virtue," so to speak, by stepping momentarily outside of her anonymous role to defend herself by emphasizing her superb intellect and thus her qualifications as a writer.

The impulse to valorize a "coming-out" by such a remarkable woman is perhaps unavoidable. But does Roland's apparent eagerness to highlight her talents contradict the restrictions she had set on publishing her writing before she was exposed? Along with Outram, commentators such as Mary Trouille and Elizabeth MacArthur have responded to this question in the affirmative. MacArthur uses the term "internalization," as does Outram, to describe a Roland who is psychologically "freed" by her imprisonment, by her expulsion from "the republic of virtue": "She has been aware all along that the political models she so admired were only for men to imitate, but she has internalized them nonetheless."[20] Trouille sees Roland as more in control of her self-image, in that she was already engaged in transforming Rousseau's "cult of domesticity" into an "empowering discourse" when the Revolution gave her the opportunity to subvert further Rousseau's dictums. Yet Trouille ultimately views Roland as an "androgynous" figure who wore a feminine "mask," and was, most tellingly, confused about her gender identity: "Above all, Mme Roland was a victim of long-standing tensions within herself between the Rousseauian ideals of domestic happiness and female self-effacement and an irresistible urge to develop her talents to the fullest—an urge that impelled her, almost in spite of herself, to take an active part in the intellectual and political life of her period."[21]

My argument is not with the contradictions critics have sketched concerning Roland's cultural situation, nor do I view her as beyond frustration with or confusion about her society's gendered norms. I am rather interested in countering the tone of confusion and sense of victimization attributed to Roland's authorial voice. Above all, I draw no clear-cut distinction between Roland's pre- and

---

[20]   Elizabeth MacArthur, "Between the Republic of Virtue and the Republic of Letters: Marie-Jeanne Roland Practices Rousseau," *Yale French Studies* 92 (1997), 196.

[21]   Mary Seidman Trouille, "Revolution in the Boudoir: Mme Roland's Subversion of Rousseau's Feminine Ideals," *Eighteenth-Century Life* 13.2 (May 1989), 81.

post-imprisonment attitudes toward women and publication. MacArthur points out that, despite her many denials, Roland was "already a writer" before she entered prison, but while she had certainly written a prolific number of "works," she was by no means an "author." The one piece published during her lifetime was shrouded in an anonymity she went to great pains to ensure. The work, a selection from her *Voyage to Switzerland*, appeared in 1788 in a short-lived magazine published by a family friend, M. Delandine.[22] In the letter Roland wrote to Delandine's wife begging her to convince her husband not to include identifying initials after the essay, Roland declares herself horrified that Delandine has apparently mistaken her wish to remain unknown as merely a feminine coyness.[23]

Roland's pre-prison relationship to public authorship was, in other words, identical to her religious practices. She wrote with furious intensity as a "private" woman. She valued her writings no less for being published in another's name, or anonymously, or not at all—during her lifetime. As Françoise Kermina notes of Roland's letters to her childhood friend, Sophie, the latter well understood that her role as a correspondent was to preserve her friend's letters for posterity, and she was careful to do so, passing them on to her son at her death.[24] I therefore disagree somewhat with MacArthur when she states that despite circulating her writings within her private circle and allowing anonymous publication, "Roland did, nevertheless, strive to conform to Rousseau's ideal for female virtue up until her imprisonment" (198). Roland's choices were not based on the internalized conviction that women should not participate in the republic of letters. The *Private Memoir* makes it clear that only a foolish woman would publish her works in such an environment of condemnation of female authorship, and Roland is far from a foolish woman: "I noticed quite early on that a woman only gains this title [author] by losing much of what she had already acquired. Men do not like her at all and her own sex criticizes her" (304). When a friend says to her that in spite of herself she will end up creating a work, she replies: "Then it will be under another's name ... for I would chew off my fingers before allowing myself to become an author" (321).

It would be difficult to argue that Roland was wrong in her assumptions, given her social standing and the cultural situation in which she found herself. That she was nevertheless hopeful that change might occur for women in the future, however minimal, is obvious in her essay on women's education from 1777, written in response to a call from the Académie de Besançon for considerations of the question "How women's education might contribute to make men better." Roland's essay—submitted, of course, anonymously—contains a mass of humble rhetorical formulations, beginning with the epigraph: "Feeling is my guide; may it take the place of wit and talent." That the author has no reason to be humble about her intellectual qualifications quickly becomes evident. In addressing male passion

---

[22]   Delandine published "Le Conservateur" in Lyons for only two years, 1787 and 1788; see *Lettres*, II:10, note 2. Roland's piece is found in *Lettres*, II:14–95.

[23]   Letter of 7 May 1788, in *Lettres*, II:11.

[24]   Kermina, *Madame Roland*, 46.

in the natural state, Roland gives an anthropological reading of the development of sentiment in human society: "Man, robust and daring, carried away by his desires, violent in his manner of satisfying them, would he ever have known pity if love had not introduced it into his heart?" In an important reformulation of Rousseau's *Discourse on Inequality*, Roland attributes the origins of pity in man to woman's influence. Whereas love is absent from natural man's repertoire for Rousseau, in which he knows only pity, and love is coexistent with pity for Laclos in the raw state of nature, however temporary its existence in men and women, Roland has love precede pity and give rise to it—but only in the presence of and under the influence of woman. Like Thomas and many others before and after her, she argues that if one casts a glance back over the course of history one sees that the respectful treatment of women can be used as a precise indication of a society's mores. Consider, she continues, in a clear sign that she has studied her sources, the "generous Germans"—those Frankish ancestors—in whose society women "enjoyed considerable distinction, acquired by the greatest fidelity to their duty."[25]

Roland also follows the standard line in declaring that women are not to be educated as strenuously as men, due to a physical weakness clearly affecting the female brain: "Abstract ideas and the solving of great problems are equally foreign to women's weak constitutions; everything that demands a powerful effort or profound thought is not within their capabilities" (460). They must be taught that their role is to be ideal wives and mothers. This role requires above all knowledge of human nature, that is to say, of morality. It follows that unless young women are students of the moral makeup of humankind ("the feminine science *par excellence*"), they will be unprepared to rear the "incomplete" moral beings known as children. What such studies might comprise is left unstated, but that such an "education" would require at least some reading and reflection is clear: "A great man has already remarked that a learned woman is a plague upon her husband and her household; I believed that an ignorant woman who is silly and frivolous is no less of a plague" (470).

As always with Roland's writings, we must consider the audience. She was capable of adopting the most conservative attitudes when the occasion seemed to call for such, a stance that is not in any sense to be construed as "hypocrisy," but rather as her moral duty to adjust her public behavior according to current standards. In prison, as she began to face the real possibility of execution, Roland's rhetoric becomes understandably more passionate: "If those who penetrated me had judged the facts for what they are, they would have spared me a sort of celebrity that I never sought" (305). The choice of the verb "to penetrate" is powerful and revealing, and brings us back again to the body. Roland's exposure as a writing woman is something of a public rape, for which she is no more

---

[25]   Marie-Jeanne Roland, *Discours, sur la question proposée par une Académie, Comment l'éducation des femmes pourrait contribuer à rendre les hommes meilleurs*, in *Lettres en partie inédites de madame Roland (mademoiselle Phlipon) aux demoiselles Cannet*, ed. Charles-Aimé Dauban (Paris: Henri Plon, 1867), II:462.

responsible than for the abuse she had suffered at the hands of the apprentice. The relationship between publishing works for the public and offering one's body for public consumption is touched on elsewhere in the *Private Memoir*, for as Outram points out, Roland's description of an aging woman novelist, Mme Benoît, is close to that of a prostitute.

This image takes on striking force when placed next to the passage I have just cited. Once beautiful, we are told, Benoît still seeks "successes" and obtains them by an ardent gaze that does not go long unanswered: "Her eyes solicited [men] with such ardor, her chest, always exposed up to that little rose whose flower is ordinarily reserved for private worship, beat so rapidly to obtain them, that it was really quite necessary to give her what she wanted" (280–81). In reacting to Roland's undeniably nasty portrait of Mme Benoît, rather than referring to authorial anxiety about notions of chastity, as does Outram, I would again refer to Roland's insistence that a woman must conform to a certain standard in public. She must, for example, take care to keep her nipples tucked into her dress, just as she would be foolish to allow her writing to be displayed if she cares a whit for her reputation. Roland was no prude about such things in general; she apparently delighted in the lack of self-consciousness exhibited by Jean-Baptiste Greuze when he took particular pains to draw her attention to his "Broken Jug," in which a young girl's recently uncovered "flower" is displayed for all to see. Anita Brookner notes that Roland apparently found the painting "a remarkably decent work."[26]

However harsh, Roland's treatment of the aging Mme Benoît is in perfect, judgmental conformity with her own notions of what must be kept private and what can be made public, when one is a woman and a writer. And possessed of an ample bosom, a trait Benoît shares with Roland, as we learn in the portrait in words she has already given, placed shortly after she experiences her first menstrual period. She has waited until after puberty, for her readings would have informed her that a person's temperament, as reflected in her physical appearance, is not fixed until that point, although she casually refers to its placement: "The moment has perhaps come to give my portrait; I might as well put it here as elsewhere. At the age of fourteen, like today, I was about five feet tall, and fully grown." She stresses the grace of her body's bearing, "firm and gracious," her "wide and superbly furnished chest," and the "open, frank, lively, and sweet look" of the eye, that "varies in its expression just like the affectionate soul whose reactions it paints; serious and proud, it at times astonishes, but it more often caresses and always awakens." She also mentions the "y-shaped veins" in her open forehead, that light up "at the slightest emotion." The presence of visible veins in her face reflects her era's obsession with these signs of humoral health in women, and she completes her portrait with an implicit reference to her sanguine body type:

---

[26]   Anita Brookner, *Greuze: The Rise and Fall of an Eighteenth-Century Phenomenon* (Greenwich, CT: New York Graphic Society, 1972), 73, 117.

> My bright complexion was very white, with brilliant colors, frequently deepened
> by a sudden reddening brought on by blood excited to a boil by the most sensitive
> of nerves; soft skin, round arms, hands pleasingly small, for my long and slender
> fingers signaled dexterity but also grace, healthy and straight teeth, a fullness
> of body indicative of perfect health, such were the treasures which a bountiful
> nature had given me. (254)

Roland's pre-Revolutionary obsession with Swiss physiognomist Johann Kaspar Lavater's theories of character also illuminates the meaning of this portrait, and explains the extreme detail into which she enters concerning her facial features: "As for my chin, which turns up, it had precisely the characteristics indicative of voluptuousness, according to the physiognomists. When I consider myself in this regard, I doubt that anyone was more suited to voluptuousness and experienced less of it." Lavater became a well-known name throughout Europe following the publication of his *Essays on Physiognomy; for the Promotion of the Knowledge and Love of Mankind* (first published in German, 1775–1778). The Roland's visited Lavater in Switzerland in 1787, on the trip that inspired Roland's *Voyage*. In her account of this meeting, Roland equates the intensity of her enthusiasm for Lavater to that of her youthful passion for Rousseau. That the former is clearly now preferable is given to be a reflection of her increased maturity of mind: "In my youthful enthusiasm, I believed that one could not be a good person and dislike the works of Jean-Jacques. In the calm state brought by age and reflection, I believed that if one is upright and sensitive of soul, one cannot know Lavater without revering and loving him."[27]

Lavaterian theory is perhaps most significant to the *Private Memoir* in that it mirrors the constant play in the autobiography between that which must remain hidden and that which can be revealed. While physiognomy allows for the "penetration" of one's secret nature against one's will, Lavater insisted that an individual had the potential to overcome his or her natural inclinations by the stoical application of willpower. Roland's self-portrait emphasizes both her innate sensuality and the contrast such indications exhibit with her simple, virtuous lifestyle. Her mouth is perhaps the most revealing of her facial features, in this respect, for the mouth is an all-important feature for Lavater. That Roland's mouth is "a bit large" reflects her chin's message of sensuality, according to Lavater's *Essay*: "Well-defined, large, and proportionate lips, the middle line of which is equally serpentine, on both sides, and easy to be drawn, though they may denote an inclination to pleasure, are never seen in a bad, mean, common, false, crouching, vicious countenance," unless excessive, for "very fleshy lips must ever have to contend with sensuality and indolence."[28]

---

[27]   Roland, *Voyage en Suisse en 1787* (Geneva: Slatkine, 1989), 90. The Roland's continued to correspond with Lavater after their visit.

[28]   John Caspar Lavater [Johann Kaspar], *Essays on Physiognomy; for the Promotion of the Knowledge and Love of Mankind*, 2nd ed., 3 vols (London: C. Whittingham, 1804), III:394.

The notion of *sensibilité* was tightly connected to the vitalist vision of human character, for it was the quality of the nervous system and the Bordelian "cellular tissue" that produced the corresponding subtlety of mind and heightened sympathy that a superior individual was believed to possess. That this quality might come dangerously close to pathology has been studied at length by Anne Vila, and indeed, in the physiological works of the period, women seem to be in a constant state of quasi-pathology. Two incidents in Roland's *Private Memoir* highlight her highly sensitive, indeed almost hysterical tendencies during her youth. First, she had to be carried to the altar by a nun to receive her first communion, so *enflammée* was her imagination, so *attendri* her heart; the nuns are said to have been suitably impressed. Second, she attempts to "breathe in death" by kissing her mother's corpse, then falls into a two-week-long state of near-catatonia (several young men are said to have noticed admiringly). Taken to the countryside to recover, she is drawn back into life only by her first reading of *The New Heloise*, given to her by "a wise and sensible man of the church." What we should grasp from these scenes is that their author was in her youth unable to control her responses to the powerful feelings inspired in her by extreme sensations. Maturity would bring with it this ability, we are to understand. When Roland finally met the man capable of inspiring true "passion" in her, she was able, she tells us in the *Private Memoir*, to resist an adulterous liaison with him. It is this resistance to acting on her highly sensual nature that makes all the difference between herself and Mme Benoît.

The fate of other Revolutionary heroines also illuminates Roland's relationship to sexuality as she so carefully crafted it. What to do about women like Roland was clearly a public relations problem for Revolutionary authorities, for a gender ideology based on the restriction of women to the private sphere in the roles of daughters, wives, and mothers was challenged when a woman became a public figure. The vilification of Queen Marie-Antoinette was a relatively simple, if nasty matter, given that she was both related to the Austrian enemy and associated with the decadence of Versailles.[29] Controlling the response to other women in the public eye could be far more complex. Such was the case for Marie-Anne-Charlotte de Corday d'Armont, who on 13 July 1793, at the age of 25, stabbed and killed Jean-Paul Marat in his wooden-shoe shaped tub, in the process going from complete obscurity to great notoriety in a matter of hours (after the rumors that a man dressed as a woman had committed the crime died out). From the Jacobin point of view, Corday was a made-to-order villainess. She had killed the self-proclaimed "friend of the people," whose constituency included the redoubtable sans-culottes. There was no question as to her guilt, for she was seized immediately following her crime at the murder scene and made no attempt to deny her guilt. Had the crowd outside been successful in seizing her and rendering the street justice for which it clamored, the story would have

---

[29] See for example Chantal Thomas, *La Reine scélérate: Marie-Antoinette dans les pamphlets* (Paris: Seuil, 1989).

ended cleanly, but Corday was successfully escorted to prison and her writings, demeanor, and actions from that point on made her a popular heroine of the most unlikely sort.

The cultural significance of Corday's fame for present-day critics lies primarily in what the vagaries of her public image reveal about the Jacobin and counter-Revolutionary propaganda machines, as well as the gendering of Revolutionary politics. As many cultural historians have noted, at the heart of the public fascination with Corday following her crime was the contradiction inherent in such a violent act having been planned and carried out by a young woman who appeared to have been otherwise a model of feminine behavior. Corday was not one of the standard Revolutionary "furies," one of the bloodthirsty *tricoteuses* supposedly calling for blood at the foot of the guillotine. She was a demure young lady who had received an excellent education for a woman of her time and social status. She was also well informed about the political situation of the day and held quite determined opinions as to the fatal course taken by the Revolution, as is clear from her trial transcript among other documents.

Guillaume Mazeau has recently published a study of the existing records concerning Corday's arrest, trial, and execution, with a view to uncovering the facts underlying the cultural myth of Marat's assassination. Mazeau notes that Corday transformed her trial from the usual spectacle of proof and denunciation met by tears and denials by the accused into a platform for the declaration of her own political views. Her audience was in other words not the judges she faced but rather the large, fascinated public present at her trial, including journalists eager to sell papers. She cut short the testimony of the first witness with "I am the one who killed him," and later undermined the prosecutor's attempt to get at her motives with her famous: "I killed one man to save a hundred thousand others."[30] Corday's defense became a prosecution of the government and her decision to assassinate one of its representatives a reaction to its delegitimization. Her testimony refers at several points to the "state of anarchy" that she knew to have taken hold in Paris.

Corday was also careful to take sole responsibility for the murder, in order to avoid implicating others, including her family members. The Revolutionary newspapers printed her trial testimony, including two letters written during her imprisonment and read aloud during the trial. One letter was addressed to Charles Jean Marie Barbaroux, one of the proscribed Girondin deputies who had taken refuge in Caen (Barbaroux had been a close friend of the Roland's), while the other was written to her father and contained an apology for having dared to "dispose of her existence" without his permission. As Mazeau notes, Corday's goal in writing her letters was to transform her cell into a *lieu de mémoire* as defined by Pierre Nora: a space of privilege in the collective memory of the French people.[31]

---

[30]   Guillaume Mazeau, *Le Bain de l'histoire: Charlotte Corday et l'attentat contre Marat 1793–2009* (Seyssel: Champ Vallon, 2009), 152–3.

[31]   Corday, "Adresse au peuple," appendix to Mazeau, *Le Bain de l'histoire*, 204.

The letter to her father, for example, plays on her ambiguity: she is a virtuous daughter apologizing for having acted without her father's permission, but the act in question is far from the type of banal transgression one would expect of a dutiful daughter filled with filial devotion.[32] Her striking lack of repentance for having committed murder was similarly offset by an utter lack of concern for her own survival. She remained calm, collected, and dignified—by all accounts the model young woman—even as she was carted off to the guillotine and publicly executed. Her "Address to the French People," also written in prison but not printed, turns her willingness to die into a useful martyrdom: "O my homeland, your misfortunes tear at my heart, I have only my life to offer you, and I praise Heaven that I am at liberty to dispose of it for you."[33]

According to Corday's letter to Barbaroux, this "Address" and Corday's overall public performance were not planned in advance of the crime. She had intended, she writes, to kill Marat and die on the spot, anonymously. She had left a letter to her father, she explains, in which she claimed to have left for England out of fear of a bloody civil war in France. Marat's illness however had confined him to his apartment, and while she regrets having used a "perfidious lie" to get close to him, "all methods are good in such a circumstance."[34] As to how a young woman could have committed such an act, her trial testimony reads: "I was a republican before the Revolution; and I have never lacked energy." Asked what she means by this last term she replies: "The resolution of those who put their particular concerns aside, and are able to sacrifice themselves for their country."[35]

Two opposing versions of Corday quickly developed, in accordance with Revolutionary and counter-Revolutionary iconography, with the latter dominating. The counter-Revolutionary Corday was beautiful, virtuous, possessed of a soft, "pleasing" voice, and yet also quite obviously guilty of a violent act—an oxymoron encapsulated in Lamartine's expression "the angel of assassination" (*History of the Girondins*, 1847). Corday's violence was presented as a transcendent moment made possible by her somewhat unearthly virtue, in other words. It helped that she was unmarried and thus a virgin, or more properly a virago, with all this term's connotations of physically Amazonian qualities subtracted. In André Chenier's "Ode to Marie-Anne-Charlotte Corday," he presents her as stepping in to fill the void created in her degenerate society by the weakness of the men who surround her—those womanly, semen-deprived eunuchs, capable neither of the physical strength necessary to wield a knife nor the moral fortitude needed to avenge Marat's victims:

---

[32] The letter is reproduced in Henri d'Almeras, *Charlotte Corday d'après les documents contemporains* (Paris: Annales, 1910), 196.

[33] Corday, "Adresse au peuple," appendix to Mazeau, *Le Bain de l'histoire*, 385.

[34] Almeras, *Charlotte Corday*, 384–5.

[35] Almeras, *Charlotte Corday*, 209.

> You alone were a man, and avenged the human race.
> And we, vile eunuchs, a cowardly, soulless herd,
> We repeat our womanly complaints,
> But the steel would weigh too heavily in our debilitated hands.[36]

While Corday's composed demeanor en route to her execution is supposed to have turned the crowd in her favor, it was the aftermath of her execution that made her a legend. According to one of the most lugubrious of Revolutionary myths, Corday maintained her exquisite feminine sensibility beyond the moment of decapitation, for her severed head was said to have "blushed" when slapped by Legros, one of the executioner's employees (Legros was put in prison for the offence).[37] In addition to giving birth to the belief that the decapitated heads of the guillotine's victims lived on for some (however short) time after being severed from the body, this further "proof" of Corday's moral virtue—expressed in the most physically horrific manner—added to her growing personal myth. She had imagined a different although equally lugubrious role for her severed head in her "Address to the French People": "may my head be carried through Paris as a rallying sign for the friends of laws."[38]

As Michael Marrinan has explored in his historical overview of Corday imagery, the minutes of the 21 January 1793 meeting of the Conseil-Général of the Département de Paris reflect the need to quash the growing worship of Corday by journalists.[39] Marrinan also quotes from an article from the *Gazette de France Nationale* designed to undermine the growing Corday worship:

> Charlotte Corday was 25 years old, which is, according to our customs, almost an old maid, the more so with her mannish carriage and tomboyish stature ... her head was full of books of every sort; she declared, or rather she avowed with an affectation which approached the ridiculous, that she had read everything, from *Tacitus* to *Portier des Chartreux*; a worthy *philosophiste*, she was without shame and modesty, and even at the trial she let it be known in her testimony that she wanted to be seen as above the childishness of her sex ... this woman absolutely threw herself outside her sex; when nature recalled her there, she experienced only disgust and boredom; sentimental love and its soft emotions no longer approach the heart of the woman who has the pretention to knowledge, to wit, to free-thought, to the politics of nations ... their tastes and their habits soon degenerate into extravagance and pretended philosophical liberty ... Charlotte Corday is a remarkable example of the seal of reprobation with which nature

---

[36]   André Chenier, "Ode à Marie-Anne-Charlotte Corday," in *Oeuvres complètes* (Paris: Gallimard, 1958), 180.

[37]   See, for example, Chapter 7 of Outram, *The Body and the French Revolution*.

[38]   Corday, "Adresse au peuple," appendix to Mazeau, *Le Bain de l'histoire*, 385.

[39]   Michael Marrinan, "Images and Ideas of Charlotte Corday: Texts and Contexts of an Assassination," *Arts Magazine* 54.8 (April 1980), 160.

stamps those women who renounce the temperament, the character, the duties, the tastes and the inclinations of their sex.[40]

The idea that the convent-educated Corday, with her strong sense of publicity, would have been so foolish as to have "avowed" reading the scandalously pornographic *Doorman of the Chartreux* is of course ridiculous. The goal is to present Corday as a degenerate, physically and morally, who has taken on male characteristics due to her reading of forbidden books. She has "renounced" feminine virtues and thus denatured herself, as her unmarried state illustrates.

The accusation of illicit promiscuity could just as easily have been made, as is evident in the persistent rumor that the authorities had Corday's body autopsied in order to prove that she was not a virgin at her death (in keeping with another of her nicknames, "the virgin of the knife").[41] The most implausible aspect of this rumor is the report that the examiner found her to be "intact," for it seems most unlikely that this unfortunate result would have been allowed.[42] The best solution to the "Corday problem" was that found by Jacques-Louis David, in his famous depiction of her crime, indeed perhaps his most famous work of art. David reduces Corday to a signature on a note in Marat's hand, for she is of course otherwise absent from "Marat Assassinated" (1793).[43] Other artists chose to emphasize her bloodthirstiness and virility, and to change her brown hair to blond, perhaps an indication that it is powdered and thus a reference to her family's nobility.[44]

Corday was active in constructing even these artistic representations. Mazeau observes: "She began working actively on her posthumous reputation the day after her arrest: for example, she asked the Comité de Sûreté générale that her portrait be made."[45] The letter containing this request is certainly calculated to make the portrait seem of interest to the Comité, for Corday notes dispassionately that "just

---

[40] As cited by Marrinan, "Images and Ideas of Charlotte Corday," 160–61; from Almeras, *Charlotte Corday*, 244–5.

[41] Mazeau does not comment on the virginity rumor, but he does declare rumors of the examination of Corday's body at the Hôpital de la Charité to be "plausible," although he found no mention of the exam in the records (*Le Bain de l'histoire*, 163–4).

[42] This theory is proposed by Almeras, *Charlotte Corday*, 234–5.

[43] See Marrinan's revealing discussion of this painting in "Images and Ideas," 161–2. Marrinan observes that the title David gave the painting was "Marat Dying," and that the painter clearly avoided any indication that we are looking at a corpse.

[44] For an analysis of the significance of this fluctuating color, see Nina Rattner Gelbart, "The Blonding of Charlotte Corday," *Eighteenth-Century Studies* 38:1 (Fall 2004), 201–21. Gelbart notes that painters most often portrayed Corday as chestnut-haired, while writers greatly favored blond, and that this blonding "reached frenzied heights with the Nazis in the 1930s and 40s" (208). See also Chantal Thomas, "Heroism in the Feminine: The Examples of Charlotte Corday and Madame Roland," in *The French Revolution: Two Hundred Years of Rethinking* (Lubbock: Texas Tech University Press, 1989), 67–82.

[45] Guillaume Mazeau, "Le Procès Corday: retour aux sources," *Annales historiques de la Révolution française* 343 (January–March 2006), 66.

as one cherishes the images of Good Citizens, curiosity makes one at times seek out those of great criminals, which perpetuates the horror of their crimes."[46] The request was denied, but Corday found a solution in Jean-Jacques Hauer, a national guardsman who had come to her trial. Noticing that Hauer was sketching her, Corday turned toward him to give him a better view. He later worked on his portrait in Corday's cell, and was present when she was taken away to her execution. Mazeau notes that Hauer manipulates the learned code of easily recognizable corporeal signs from the period, including a blondeness that signifies something quite different from aristocratic degeneracy:

> Corday appears not in the least a degenerate: her blondeness and her light eyes suggest purity, her elongated nose and chin signal determination, her high forehead is a sign of intelligence, her white complexion of nobility. We contemplate a vestal, clothed in immaculate white, her hands piously placed on her knees. This painting, quickly engraved by Anselin, played in the moderate and counter-Revolutionary milieus the opposite role to David's, but three months in advance.[47]

The most persuasive treatment of Corday's place in the gendered realm of Revolutionary politics is Elizabeth R. Kindleberger's "Charlotte Corday in Text and Image." Citing Dorinda Outram, among others, Kindleberger notes the common belief that women were at this time either to remain in the private realm or to commit a transgression against the ideal of femininity, in their own eyes as much as in the public's. This ideal, Kindleberger observes, was based on a new gender system that "after straining for expression and institutionalization for more than a generation, crystallized during the Revolution with the reordering of public and private spheres."[48] Kindleberger is arguing, as I am for Roland, that there was a far more complex equation at work in Corday's public representation than has generally been recognized. She demonstrates that the combination of Corday's single act of violence with her calm demeanor and virginal beauty was far more attractive than repulsive to the French public, even during one of the most violent and repressive months of the Revolution as a whole: "Shining simultaneously with disinterested public devotion and sensual and emotional appeal ... Corday could be said to embody the triumph of revolutionary virtue over Old Regime vice for many contemporaries" (979). For Kindleberger, Corday was viewed as "eloquent *and* sensitive, civic-minded *and* a dutiful daughter," and the existence of these dichotomies proves the complexity of Revolutionary gender politics (990). Her reading of Corday is ultimately an optimistic, forward-looking analysis:

---

[46]   Almeras, *Charlotte Corday*, 182. Almeras notes that at Corday's request, Hauer sent a copy of his portrait to her family.

[47]   Mazeau, "Le Procès Corday," 67.

[48]   Elizabeth R. Kindleberger, "Charlotte Corday in Text and Image: A Case Study in the French Revolution and Women's History," *French Historical Studies* 18:4 (Fall 1994): 973. Future references in the text.

Corday's ability to portray the resolution of basic revolutionary terms by combining masculine and feminine qualities may not contradict interpretations of the transgressive Corday based on the idea of the Revolution's inscription of a new gender system, but it does complicate them. As the Revolution sought to build a new society, a 'new man,' based on well-defined gender roles, there existed a simultaneous longing to transcend that pattern, to rise above the binary tensions that structured society, thought and feeling. (979)

I would be less abstract in my reading of Corday and conclude that this particular embodiment of the "new woman"—well read, politically savvy, and able to carry out an assassination and deal with its aftermath with an amazing degree of sang-froid—was working to control her public image within this changing cultural landscape, just as Roland would do soon after in writing her *Private Memoir*. Louise Colet counts among the many who have placed Corday and Roland alongside each other as heroines, for in the preface to her play *Charlotte Corday et Mme Roland* (1842), she describes her work as "a sketch of two women, two noble figures that stand out radiantly from a bloody background."[49] Roland seems to have shared this vision of Corday, for although she was arrested before Marat's assassin, Roland was executed after her. Roland was briefly freed (a technical error led to this liberation and rearrest), and in her short piece "Second Arrest" she notes that her original cell in the Abbaye Prison would later be occupied by "a heroine worthy of a better century, the famous *Corday*" (176). She describes Corday as "an astonishing woman" who "deserves the admiration of the universe," adding that, unfortunately, she chose both her moment and her victim badly (184). Many commentators have since agreed with Roland that the result of Corday's act was to increase the vehemence of the attacks on the Girondins and to allow the relatively unimpeded rise of Robespierre—no doubt Roland's preferred victim.[50] But in the *Private Memoir*, in stressing the importance of defending the innocence of the Girondins in the matter of Marat's murder, she notes that it would be absurd to suppose that anyone could have forced this admirable young woman's hand, for no would could "command the resolution of a Corday" (361).

Roland's admiration for Corday is seemingly not affected by the violence of Marat's murder. Like Roland's own public self-defense, Corday's violent defense of a republic in danger is brought on by extreme circumstances and therefore is perhaps to be seen as in no way a violation of her "feminine" version of stoic virtue. I would not go so far as to say that Roland sought to "rise above binary tensions," given that this goal would seem to indicate an anachronistic form of

---

[49] Louise Colet, *Charlotte Corday et Mme Roland* (Paris: Berquet and Pétion, 1842), v. For a discussion of Colet's play in the context of historical representations of Corday, see Mazeau, *Le Bain de l'histoire*, 189.

[50] Mazeau overstates Roland's condemnation of Corday (*Le Bain de l'histoire*, 165, 178 note 1); Roland is quite gentle in her critique, implying that Corday was not close enough to the events of the capital to realize the complications that might ensue from her act (*Mémoires*, 184).

equality feminism quite foreign to her mentality; but I do see Roland as actively engaging the tensions in her culture in order to present herself as a highly rational yet also fully feminine woman. It is her engagement in the arguments about the nature of women that were very much in the forefront of her culture's social agenda that makes her *Private Memoir* such a fascinating and useful document. Alongside the works of the physiologists and of such cultural philosophers as Diderot, Rousseau, and Laclos, Roland's writings fully engage the attempt to build a "new woman" at the end of the eighteenth century that has been so very overshadowed by studies of the "new man." However tragic the fate of this one woman, her rhetorical struggles to define her virtue while retaining her claims to sensuality and to superior rationality are far from evidence of "internalized" notions of womanhood. Her *Private Memoir* is a record of an argument engaged not with herself, but with her readers, envisioned as both contemporary and belonging to the "impartial posterity" of the post-Revolutionary era. Roland was reacting to and participating in one of the major cultural discussions of her day: the attempt to define the nature of woman and of man as well in the wake of the two-sex model. She played as much a part as any woman could have in her era's medical revolution and was as proud of this role as she was of her influence on her country's political revolution.

Conclusion:
Sade's Way

> But, you object, there is an age at which men's actions do undoubted harm to the
> health of a young girl. This consideration is meaningless; as soon as you agree
> to the right to pleasure, this right is independent of the effects produced by that
> pursuit.

—Sade, Philosophy in the Boudoir

Any study of sexual enlightenment and cultural degradation in eighteenth-century
France would be incomplete without a reference to the writer who most fully
embraced these two concepts in his work, and not, of course, in a negative sense:
Donatien Alphonse François, Marquis de Sade. Undoing a convent education by
convincing young girls that they should seek sexual pleasure without reserve is the
central theme of such famous Sadeian texts as *Justine or the Misfortunes of Virtue*
(1791) and *Philosophy in the Boudoir or the Immoral Teachers* (1795). As for
cultural "degradation," the main problem with eighteenth-century French society,
as Sade hyperbolically portrays it, is that young French men and women are kept
from engaging in the types of activities labeled "dangerous" or "perverting" by
the religious authorities and medical professionals. If these promising young
specimens are to grow into the strong libertines that "nature" intends them to be,
they must learn Her lessons early and put them into practice often.

For Sade, a strong culture is comprised of strong individuals—with the fate
of the weak, not to mention the future of the "race," a non-issue. As is argued in
the epigraph above, should the sexual desires of the dominant members of society
clash with the health of an individual—in this instance, a young prepubescent
girl—the pleasure given to the strong, adult man more than makes up for the
damage done to the object of his desire. In other words, although Sade was
certainly aware of the physiologists' writings on sexuality, he would have no
person, of whatever age or stage of development, exempted from the necessity
of submitting to the sexual caprices of others. The extent of Sade's knowledge
of the biological sciences of his day has been explored by Jean Duprun, who
emphasizes the importance of electricity to Sadeian physiology. Duprun explains
that by borrowing from d'Holbach and La Mettrie, Sade theorizes a materialist
soul consisting of an ethereal (electrical) fluid that by circulating in the "cavities"
of the nerves produces greater or lesser sensations in accordance with the intensity
of external forces acting upon the human body.[1] According to this physiological

---

[1]   Jean Duprun, "Sade et la philosophie biologique de son temps," in *Le Marquis
de Sade* (Paris: Armand Colin, 1968), 2. Duprun notes that Sade quotes Buffon twice in
his works.

vision, "Nature" would have us, or rather our human nature compels us, to seek out as much "soul"-stimulation as possible. Should this pursuit take place on a scale large enough to decimate the human race, no great harm would be done, for as Duprun notes, Sade also believed in the spontaneous generation of life.[2] The production and expenditure of energy—electricity, in its purest form—is the defining aspect of nature's plan, and the outcome of this wild orgy of energy for any individual human being, any society, or even the human species as a whole, is meaningless in comparison to the necessity of the continual build up and release of energy.

That nature would have humans seek the unregulated pursuit of the pleasures of human sexuality is thus the lesson that any self-respecting Sadeian character is to learn. But while Sade inverses the rules of the physiologists and the lessons of the novelist/moralists of his day, he does share one striking commonality with these two groups: his heroine of choice is the freshly minted, convent educated girl. For Sade as for the many physiologists and writers who came before him, the attraction of the ingénue lies in her liminal status. She has been awakened to sexual desire by the physical experience of puberty, but is unaware of the nature of her feelings, a combination that is both productive and highly amusing to observe. The ingénue's "vulnerability," for Sade, lies in her status as the supreme target of her society's efforts to contain female sexuality and channel its energy into monogamy and marriage. The ingénue is, for all of these reasons, the pupil of choice for Sade's eager libertine educators. While it is difficult to choose the star student of the Sadeian oeuvre, the 15-year-old Eugénie of *Philosophy in the Boudoir* is stunningly quick to adapt to her preceptors' lessons, with this alacrity to be read as proof of the "naturalness" of the libertine program. Eugénie certainly exhibits the most perverse tendencies of any Sadeian pupil during what might be said to constitute her "final exam," for she enthusiastically agrees to sew up her mother's vagina in order to contain the syphilis just deposited there by an infected valet.

The "worst" pupil of all the girl students in the Sadeian fictional universe is easy to identify: Justine. The younger sister of Juliette, one Sade's most famous libertine women characters, Justine is stubbornly unwilling to acknowledge—or incapable of acknowledging—that the experiential "misfortunes" to which she is repeatedly subjected are so many arrows pointing to the truth of Sadeian libertinism. Justine's resistance to the Sadeian lesson is more revealing than the embrace of this philosophy by his libertine heroines, and I briefly conclude my study with how Justine's misfortunes, or rather Sade's late-century, sui generis commentary on female sexuality and cultural degradation, echo eighteenth-century physiological and literary treatments of these themes.

There are three versions of Justine's story. The first, *The Misfortunes of Virtue*, was written in 1787 but never published. The second, longer novel is *Justine or the Misfortunes of Virtue* (1791), and was Sade's first published work. A third and even longer version appeared in 1799 and was given a title that is a quite obvious

---

2   Duprun, "Sade," 201.

nod to Rousseau: *The New Justine or the Misfortunes of Virtue, Followed by the Story of Juliette, Her Sister*. The basic narrative remains the same throughout the evolution of this novel, although the level of obscenity increases dramatically and the number of Justine's "misfortunes" increases exponentially with each rewriting. The details of the long list of misadventures to which the young Justine is subjected are not of interest to me; I consider instead the physiological attributes given to Justine and her sister as the story opens, then turn to the conclusion of her story, a vicious parody of the sexual "enlightenment" of young girls.

All three versions of this novel begin with a brief description of the rich, immoral, and beautiful Mme la comtesse de Lorsange—Juliette, now rich and living in all the comforts available to wealthy eighteenth-century nobles. The narrator then takes us back in time to begin Juliette and Justine's story from the beginning, that is, with the bankruptcy and death of their parents. With only 100 *écus* in their pockets and no protectors, the two girls are kicked out of the abbatial setting in which they had been living and onto the streets of Paris. But before their adventures begin, we are treated to a description of the young girls, in which Justine's age varies from text to text. Her sister Juliette is given to be 15 at the time she leaves the convent in all three versions, but while her younger sibling is said in the first version to be "a year younger" than Juliette, this statement is immediately contradicted by a reference to her age as 12. She is 12 without contradiction in the second, published version, and 14 in the third (*The New Justine*).

Another, subtler difference is to be found in the description of the girls' education, for in the *The Misfortunes of Virtue* Sade insists that Juliette/Mme de Lorsange "had received the most brilliant education ... in one of the best convents of Paris ... no advice, no master, no good book, no talent had been refused her."[3] This impressive education is extended to her sister Justine in the second version, although the denial of "no good book" to the two sisters is revised to the denial of "no book." The father who provides for this education is also switched from a wealthy "businessman" to a "rich banker," and the girls' place of residence from a mere convent to "one of the most famous Abbeys" in Paris (*Justine*, II:133). In the third and last version of the work their father, still a rich banker, has placed them again in the famous Abbey, where they are again denied "no book," rather than "no good book." We are told in this version that the two girls were the envy of all who saw them, for it seemed that "morality, religion, talents ... had formed these young persons" (*The New Justine*, II:396).

Juliette and Justine, in other words, are not fully "innocent" in the conventional, or rather conventual, sense, when they are deposited on the mean streets of eighteenth-century Paris. Their privileged lifestyle in the abbey included access to knowledge about the outside world, and the revision of "no good book" to

---

[3]   D. A. F. de Sade, *Les Infortunes de la vertu*, in *Oeuvres* (Paris: Gallimard, 1990), I:3. *Justine ou les malheurs de la vertu* and *La Nouvelle Justine ou les malheurs de la vertu* are also contained in the first volume of this nédition of Sade's collected works; future references to all three novels will be in the text.

"no book" even invites us to understand that the sisters perhaps had at their disposal novels as well as philosophical, scientific, and other texts, a reading list that would have horrified the authors of the era's hygiene treatises. Paule Constant's comment about the type of reading material contained in the convent schools of this period is telling: "There were simply no novels ... None at Port-Royal, none at Saint-Cyr, no novels at the Ursiline or the Visitandine convents, and if there were any at the Abbaye-aux-Bois, they were perhaps hidden deep within its 16,000-volume-rich library."[4] It would appear that Sade's young fictional heroines were granted access to a fictional abbey library of great richness, and although "morality and religion" may appear to have formed them, we are invited to believe that they were influenced by reading material not commonly catalogued under those rubrics.

As Sade's narrative moves on to demonstrate, the benefit either sister might have gained from having access to such works would have depended on the most important influence on their respective fates: their innate characters. Sade takes care to give us a physiological (and in the process, moral) portrait of each sister, and the two girls are a study in contrasts. While the black-haired and dark-eyed future libertine Juliette is said to possess spirit, wit, a lively intelligence, and an expression of coquettishness, the younger Justine, possessed of "the most beautiful blond hair" and "blue eyes," is described as chaste and disposed to religious piety. Judged by the ability to succeed in the Sadeian fictional universe, Juliette can thus be said to possess all the requisite characteristics. She is highly sensual, as her hair color demonstrates, and this sensuality is a fixed attribute of her temperament, for at 15, she has passed through the process of puberty and emerged a fully developed young woman. Justine, to the contrary, is only 12 (at least in the first two versions of the work), an age identified with the very beginnings of the stirrings of puberty, at the most. She is described in the first version as possessing a "somber and melancholic" character, although she is said to be also highly "sensitive" (*sensible*), an important detail, for we are to understand that she will not reject libertinism out of a merely physical insensibility, as her blondeness might otherwise indicate. Her coloration represents instead a moral "disfiguration," judged according to Sadeian standards, for she is said to be "of an ingenuousness, a candor, and a good faith that would make her fall into many traps," while the pathos of her blue eyes combined with her "virginal air" work to make her a born victim (*Misfortunes*, II:5). The importance of these physiological details is indicated by their static quality; by the third version Justine is said to be "somber and romantic" (rather than "somber and melancholic"), but she is otherwise unchanged (*The New Justine*, II:397).

When told they must soon leave the Abbey, the two sisters react according to type. Juliette looks forward to the life of freedom she is about to undertake and relies on her beauty and youth to make her way in the world; Justine, however fearful of what awaits her, is horrified by her sister's proposal that they use the physical attractions nature has given them to make their fortune. Even in the most obscene version, *The New Justine*, the older sister still attempts to prepare her

---

4   Paule Constant, *Un Monde à l'usage des demoiselles* (Paris: Gallimard, 2002), 265.

younger sibling for life beyond the abbatial walls: "Juliette wanted to wipe away her sister's tears. Seeing that she could not do so, she began to scold her for her sensitivity." She explains to Justine that it is "possible to find in oneself physical sensations of such striking voluptuousness that they extinguish all painful moral feeling"—pity for others included (*The New Justine*, II:397). One can, that is to say, experience a sensual pleasure so overpowering that it allows us to forget our moral scruples and otherworldly worries. She then proceeds (only in this third version, however) to demonstrate this "truth" to her sister by masturbating to orgasm in front of her—to Justine's horror.

Although quite obviously a born libertine pedagogue, Juliette's lesson is nevertheless wasted on her sister. Her skill is not however wasted on the narrator, who comments that this sororal lesson inside the Abbey walls was proof of "a philosophy very advanced for one of her age, and that demonstrated the most singular natural propensities" (*The New Justine*, II:397). One can assume that in addition to these natural gifts, Juliette's unrestricted reading, alongside the powerful sensations of puberty, have alerted her to the philosophical potentials of sexual activity. In the face of their mutually exclusive worldviews, the two sisters recognize that they must separate, and say their goodbyes at the door of the Abbey. Juliette pursues a brief career as a prostitute and kept woman before becoming a rich countess. Her passive, religious sister, to the contrary and in accordance with her religious enthusiasm, instead undergoes a series of humiliating and violent sexual encounters, losing her cherished virginity along the way, and yet refusing to renounce her belief in the merits of virtue no matter what the (astonishing number of) libertines she encounters do to her.

The narrator makes bitingly sarcastic asides throughout the course of this negative education, of course, many parodying not only the Church's doctrine but also the advice of the era's physiologists. At one point, as a man of the church is cruelly abusing Justine, we are told that, "should her torturer have torn her to bits, she would have never dared to complain." We are then told in an "editor's note" that this ability to suffer in silence is proof of "the extreme connection between the moral and the physical; learn to elevate the one, and you will always be master of the other: and so is explained all the enthusiasm of martyrs" (*The New Justine*, II:596). After more than driving home, especially in the third and last version, that Justine will never accept the lessons that Nature and her tireless libertines have been working to teach her, Sade finally reunites the battered Justine with the now rich and powerful Juliette, comtesse de Lorsange. Juliette takes Justine back to the castle she calls home—where her sister is struck by lightning and killed. Justine's obtuse refusal to throw aside societal proscriptions is the greatest of all philosophical crimes in Sade's works, and as a crime against the expression of sexual desire, it merits the death penalty, administered by "Nature" herself in the case of this well-hardened believer in sexual continence.

We are to understand this bolt from the sky as a forcible "enlightenment," a deus ex machina ending that demonstrates nature's wrath at Justine's obduracy. Again, there are variations in the three texts that reveal Sade's increasing efforts to make the meaning of this ironic death as clear as possible to his readers. In the first two versions of the story, this lightning bolt is said to enter through Justine's right breast. After having "consumed" her chest and her face, it leaves through her stomach, leaving the "miserable creature" horrifying to behold (*Justine*, II:388). With questionable hermeneutic skills, Juliette reads the lightning bolt as a message from God: "*The prosperity of vice* is but the test to which Providence puts virtue, *it is like lightning, the illusory fires of which momentarily embellish the atmosphere while casting the unfortunate into the abyss of hell*" (II:389).

In both *The Misfortunes of Virtue* and *Justine or the Misfortunes of Virtue*, the contemplation of this demonstration of "celestial" power causes Juliette to retire to a convent and seek forgiveness. That this dénouement is in keeping with libertine materialism, or at least with the sarcastic undoing of the moral tenets of Christianity, is argued by Michel Delon, who notes of Juliette's "improbable" conversion that "Justine suffers so that her sister, hardened by crime, may finally open her eyes and be saved in her turn."[5] Even God, it would appear, favors the older sister, who is able to enjoy her youth before saving her soul. In *The New Justine*, however, there is no divine salvation for Juliette, who remains firmly ensconced in the "Church" of Nature. In addition, the sisters' reunion is in this version the catalyst for Juliette to pick up and recite the long, long story of her life and crimes, an illustration of "the prosperities of vice" that is not upended by the novel's ending, sarcastically or otherwise. Juliette tells her tale not only to her sister but also to her libertine friends, another addition to the narrative. Her story finally finished, a storm develops and the libertines decide to engage in a "science experiment" of sorts by forcing Justine outside in order to "tempt fate." She is, of course, almost immediately hit by lightning. The libertines make the meaning of the lightning strike perfectly clear, in case the reader should be in doubt, calling out to Justine: "She is dead! ... come and contemplate the work of Heaven? come see how it rewards virtue." More to the point, Sade also makes the sexual basis of this metaphor of "enlightenment" impossible to misinterpret in this third version, for we read that "the lightning bolt, having entered by her mouth, left through her vagina"—at which point, in case we have still not entirely understood, we are told that the libertines proceed "to make horrible jokes about the two routes taken by the celestial fire" as they have their way with Justine's lifeless body. As they return to the castle, Madame de Lorsange (who has no intention of withdrawing to a convent) interprets Justine's death as the final evidence of the wisdom of her chosen path: "Oh Nature! ... it is thus a necessary part of your plan, this crime against which the fools take it upon themselves to rage; you clearly desire it, for your hand has punished, in this manner, those who fear it or refuse to give themselves over to it."[6]

Justine's inability to respond to the "specific" cure of sexual intercourse and give herself over to libertinism is to be understood above all as a narrative

---

5   Michel Delon, "Introduction" to D. A. F. de Sade, *Oeuvres*, II:xiii.

6   D. A. F. de Sade, *Histoire de Juliette*, in *Oeuvres*, III:1259.

necessity. It allows Sade to elaborate the number of "crimes" committed against her, all the while illustrating with increasing intensity the level of her obstinacy (he was working on a fourth expansion of the *Misfortunes*, seized by the police when he was arrested in 1801). As for the symbolic value of Justine's obstinate/ innate blindness with regard to her status as an "ingénue," the full meaning of her resistance becomes clear only when read in conjunction with *Philosophy in the Boudoir*, Sade's perverted take on *Emile*. At one point in this work the libertine pedagogues and their student Eugénie, exhausted by their exertions, pause to rest. To pass the time instructively, their "head master" of sorts, Dolmancé, reads a "Revolutionary pamphlet" with the exhortatory title "Yet Another Effort, Frenchmen, if You Want to Be Republicans!" This work-within-a-work teaches the reader that Justine's impermeability should be seen as an inherited illness, along the same lines as Merteuil's latent case of syphilis, albeit pointing to a far different conclusion. The pamphlet writer begins by instructing the republican reader of the need to extirpate the "germ" of religion in the new generation (the "nephews" of the Revolution), a germ said to manifest itself as "modesty" in women. We are told that "modesty, far from a virtue, was rather the first effect of corruption"—the first symptom of a societal illness, that is to say, a malady that will manifest itself in its full blown state as an insistence on monogamy.[7]

The inevitable reference to the state of nature follows. The Sadeian version of originary female sexuality is, as always, a revealingly perverted version of the commonplaces of the day. He begins by declaring that women in the state of nature were born *vulgivagues*, that is, they "belonged, like [the other female animals], and without exception, to all the males." This rule in itself constituted "the first laws of nature and the only institutions established by the first gatherings of men" (III:132). Corruption first manifests itself in the desire for exclusive possession, although rather than citing Rousseau's *Discourse* and berating the first man to enclose a piece of land, Sade echoes Laclos in declaring that a man's desire to "possess" one woman for himself was the principal cause of the decline of the human condition ("greediness, egoism, and love, degraded these first, simple, and natural principles," III:132). Sade then equates the condition of these women/ possessions with slavery, as did Laclos, in what might seem, if read in isolation, like a protofeminist declaration. This impression is undone by Sade's conclusion that women in the new Republic he envisions therefore have no right to refuse themselves to any man who desires them.[8] Force may be used should they refuse, "we" are told: "Eh! did not nature prove that we have this right, in allotting us the strength necessary to submit them to our desires?" (III:133).

---

[7] D. A. F. de Sade, *La Philosophie dans le boudoir*, in *Oeuvres*, III:130. Future references in the text.

[8] The debate over Sade and women (horrific misogynist or protofeminist?) has ranged widely, with Angela Carter arguing, most notably, in favor of the liberating potential of his writing (*The Sadeian Woman and the Ideology of Pornography* [London: Virago Press, 1979]).

The problem with this "enslavement," in other words, is not what it did to women per se, but rather the resulting removal of most women from the available pool of sexual partners. One should avoid, it almost goes without saying, taking Sade's theories of the evolution of social groups too literally or too seriously— to do so would mean quite missing the point, or at least most of the point, of Sade's tongue-in-cheek lubriciousness. I will conclude by simply casting a glance at the role of female modesty in "Frenchmen!"—that "corrupting" factor said to accompany the degradation of the primeval libertine utopia to which Sade refers as the "state of nature." It would seem that the development of female modesty is as much to blame for the perpetuation of monogamy as is the male desire to possess a woman for himself, although modesty was an outgrowth of that possessiveness. Modesty is ascribed to women in the state of nature by almost all eighteenth-century theorists of this moment in human history, Laclos included, but for Sade it is a "germ" that develops only as a result of women's "enslavement" and becomes in the process hereditary. He insists in "Frenchmen!" that it will take several generations to "cure" the nephews of the "disease" of religion, and the republican readers are encouraged to work hard at educating their progeny along these lines.

But as for the "nieces," who possess the germ of modesty in addition to the disease of religious belief, they are not to be coddled or "educated" out of their sickness over time. They are to be forcibly constrained to have sex whenever a man desires them, and this despite any damage that may be done to them, for while Sade accepts that "there is an age at which men's actions do undoubted harm to the health of a young girl," he quickly declares this consideration to be meaningless (*sans aucune valeur*). A revealing analogy immediately precedes this declaration: "He who has the right to eat the fruit of a tree may surely pick it ripe or green as his tastes direct him" (III:134). The Biblical resonance of this image is quite obvious: there is no forbidden fruit in Sade's primeval utopia, one may pick the fruit of any tree at will, be it "ripe" or not. The Bible is not the only work attacked here however, for the physiologists' prescriptions against precocious sexual behavior are equally rejected. We are to understand that Sade of course realizes that, according to the medical theories of his day, prepubescent girls are irremediably harmed by sexual intercourse: their development is disrupted, and they will never become healthy, full-grown women. Sade does not seem to be speaking of specific physical damage done to the young girl's body (tearing, etc.), for he refers to the "decided" harm done to her "health" (*santé*) at a certain age. We remember that Eugénie, like Juliette before her, is 15 when she is first "enlightened" as to the pleasures of heterosexual intercourse (Mme de Saint-Ange had, Merteuil-like, introduced Eugénie to the pleasures of physical sensation in the convent, but these experiments are not accorded any more "enlightening" power in Sade than they carry in *Dangerous Liaisons*). Justine's "misfortunes" may well have had their physiological basis in more than her blond hair and blue eyes; she is given to be 12 in the first two versions of her tale, an age that would have made her the equivalent of the Sadeian "green fruit." By the third version, however, at age 14, the "new" Justine is to be understood as simply obstinate, and more than deserving of the death Nature sends her.

Ultimately, of course, Sade's libertines are free to destroy the human race as a whole (along with their unborn children, if they are women) in order to ensure the continuing engorgement and exquisite expulsion of the electrical desires flowing through their veins. Perhaps above all in his willingness to include the extinction of the human race as a natural outcome of Nature's design, Sade's work can be read as an inverted compendium of eighteenth-century views on the necessity of regulating female sexual desire through enforced ignorance and the encouragement of "natural" female modesty in young girls. The "dangerous" force of sexual desire, born of the exquisitely painful "engorgement" of puberty, is in no need of regulation, in the Sadeian fictional universe. If read as so many inversions of the commonplaces of his day, Sade's unique declarations concerning female sexuality in the state of nature and in the ideal civilized society are grounded in the presuppositions of the novels and medical treatises explored in the previous chapters. Whether as Marquis (*The Misfortunes of Virtue*, 1787) or Citizen (*Philosophy in the Boudoir*, 1795), Sade put forward a twisted, often intentionally comic version of the mind–body link that dominated the philosophical and medical theories of young womanhood from mid-century on.

Works Cited

Primary Sources

Almeras, Henri de. *Charlotte Corday d'après les documents contemporains*. Paris: Annales, 1910.

Astruc, Jean. *Traité des Maladies des femmes*. 6 vols. Paris: Cavelier, 1761–1765.

Ballexserd, Jacques. *Dissertation sur l'Education physique des enfans, Depuis leur naissance jusqu'à l'âge de puberté*. Paris: Vallat-La-Chappelle, 1762.

Berquin, Arnaud. *L'Ami des enfants*. 12 vols. London: Elmsley, 1782–1783.

Bienville, J. D. T. *De La Nymphomanie ou Traité de la fureur utérine*. Amsterdam: Marc-Michel Rey, 1771.

Bordeu, Antoine de, Théophile de Bordeu, and François de Bordeu. *Recherches sur les maladies chroniques*. Paris: Ruault, 1775.

Bordeu, Théophile de. *Recherches anatomiques sur la position des glandes et sur leur action*. Paris: Quillau Père, 1751.

———. *Recherches sur quelques points de l'histoire de la médecine*. Liège/Paris: Cailleau, 1764.

———. *Recherches sur le tissu muqueux, ou l'organe cellulaire, et sur quelques maladies de la poitrine*. Paris: Didot le jeune, 1767.

Boy, Simon. *Abrégé sur les maladies des femmes grosses, et de celles qui sont accouchées ... et la manière de soigner et traiter les enfans, depuis la naissance jusques vers l'âge de puberté*. Paris: Croullebois, 1788.

Bressy, Joseph. *Recherches sur les vapeurs*. Paris: Planche, 1789.

Buffon, George-Louis Leclerc, comte de. *Histoire naturelle, générale et particulière, avec la description du cabinet du roi*. 36 vols. Paris: Imprimerie Royale, 1749–1788.

Cabanis, P. J. G. [Pierre-Jean-Georges]. *Rapports du physique et du moral de l'homme*. 2 vols. Paris: Crapart, Caille, and Ravier: An X [1802].

Charrière, Isabelle de. *Lettres de Mistriss Henley publiées par son amie*. Ed. Joan Hinde Stewart and Philip Stewart. New York: Modern Language Association, 1993.

Chenier, André. *Oeuvres complètes*. Ed. Gérard Walter. Paris: Gallimard, 1958.

Condorcet, Jean-Antoine-Nicolas de Caritat, marquis de. *Esquisse d'un tableau historique des progrès de l'esprit humain*. Ed. Yvon Belaval and O. H. Prior. Paris: Vrin, 1970.

Daignan, Guillaume. *Tableau des variétés de la vie humaine, avec les avantages et les désavantages de chaque constitution et des avis très-importans aux pères et aux mères sur la santé de leurs enfants, de l'un & de l'autre sexe, sur-tout à l'âge de puberté*. 2 vols. Paris: Chez l'Auteur, 1786.

Démeunier, Jean-Nicolas. *L'Esprit des usages et des coutumes des différens peuples*. Paris: Pissot, 1776.

Desessartz, Jean-Charles. *Traité de l'éducation corporelle des enfants en bas âge ou Réflexions pratiques sur les moyens de procurer une meilleure constitution aux citoyens*. Paris: Herissant, 1760.

Diderot, Denis. *Oeuvres*. Ed. André Billy. Paris: Gallimard, 1951.

Dusoulier, P. *Avis aux jeunes gens des deux sexes*. Angers: Mame, 1810.

Encyclopédie ou Dictionnaire raisonné des sciences, des arts et des métiers. Ed. Denis Diderot and Jean d'Alembert. 17 vols. Paris: Briasson, [etc.], 1751–1772. University of Chicago: ARTFL Encyclopédie Project. Spring 2011 Edition. Ed. Robert Morrissey. http://encyclopedie.uchicago.edu/.

Ferrier, P. M. [Paul]. *De la Puberté considérée comme crise des maladies de l'enfance. Collection des thèses soutenues à l'école de médecine de Montpellier, en l'an VII*. Montpellier: Tournel, an VII [1799].

Goulin, Jean. *Le Médecin des dames, ou l'Art de les conserver en santé*. Paris: Vincent, 1771.

———. *Le Médecin des hommes, depuis la puberté jusqu'à l'extrême vieillesse*. Paris: Vincent, 1772.

Guarinoni, Hippolyt. *Die Grewel der Verwuüstung menschlichen Geschlechts*. Ingolstatt: Angermayr, 1610.

La Caze, Louis de. *Idée de l'homme physique et moral, pour servir d'Introduction à un Traité de Médecine*. Paris: Guérin and Delatour, 1755.

La Fontaine, Jean de la. *Oeuvres complètes*. Ed. René Groos and Jacques Schiffrin. 2 vols. Paris: Gallimard, 1954, 1958.

Laclos, Choderlos de. *Oeuvres complètes*. Ed. Laurent Versini. Paris: Gallimard, 1979.

———. *Les Liaisons dangereuses*. Ed. Catriona Seth. Paris: Gallimard, 2011.

Lavater, John Caspar [Johann Kaspar]. *Essays on Physiognomy; for the Promotion of the Knowledge and Love of Mankind*. Trans. Thomas Holcroft. 2nd ed. 3 vols. London: C. Whittingham, 1804.

[Le Camus, Antoine]. *Abdeker, ou l'Art de préserver la beauté*. L'an de l'Hegyre 1168 [Paris, 1754].

Le Moré, Abbé. *Principes d'institution ou de la manière d'élever les enfans des deux sexes, par rapport au corps, à l'esprit et au coeur*. Paris: La Veuve Desaint, 1774.

Le Rebours, Marie-Angélique Anel. *Avis aux mères qui veulent nourrir leurs enfants*. Utrecht, Paris, 1767.

L***[Lignac], M. [Louis François Luc] de. *De l'Homme et de la femme considérés physiquement dans l'état de mariage*. 2 vols. Lille: J. B. Henry, 1772.

Ménuret de Chambaud, Jean-Jacques. *Avis aux mères sur la petite vérole et la rougeole*. Lyons: Frères Périsse, 1769.

Montesquieu, Charles de Secondat, baron de. *Oeuvres complètes*. Ed. Roger Caillois. 2 vols. Paris: Gallimard, 1949, 1951.

Moreau de la Sarthe, Louis-Jacques. *Histoire naturelle de la femme*. 3 vols. Paris: Duprat, Letellier, 1803.

Plutarch. *Moralia*. 15 vols. Cambridge, MA: Harvard University Press, 1949–1976.

Pomme, Pierre. *Essai sur les Affections vaporeuses des deux sexes*. Paris: Desaint and Saillant, 1760.

Prévost, Antoine-François, abbé de. *Histoire du chevalier Des Grieux et de Manon Lescaut*. Ed. Maurice Allem. Paris: Garnier, 1952.

Raciborski, M. A. [Adam]. *De la puberté et de l'âge critique chez la femme*. Paris: Baillière, 1844.

Raulin, Joseph. *De la conservation des enfans, Ou les moyens de les fortifier, de les préserver & guérir des maladies, depuis l'instant de leur existence, jusqu'à l'âge de puberté*. Paris: Merlin, 1749.

———. *Traité des fleurs blanches*. Paris: Herissant, 1766.

Riccoboni, Marie-Jeanne. *Oeuvres*. 9 vols. Paris, Brissot-Thivars, 1826.

Roland, Marie-Jeanne. *Oeuvres de J. M. Ph. Roland, Femme de l'ex-ministre de l'intérieur*. Ed. L. A. Champagneux. 3 vols. Paris: Bidault, an VIII [1800].

———. *Lettres en partie inédites de madame Roland (mademoiselle Phlipon) aux demoiselles Cannet*. Ed. Charles-Aimé Dauban. 2 vols. Paris: Plon, 1867.

———. *Lettres de Madame Roland*. Ed. Claude Perroud. 2 vols. Paris: Imprimerie Nationale, 1900–1902.

———. *Mémoires de Mme Roland*. Ed. Paul de Roux. Paris: Mercure de France, 1986.

———. *Voyage en Suisse en 1787*. Geneva: Slatkine, 1989.

Rousseau, Jean-Jacques. *Oeuvres complètes*. Ed. Bernard Gagnebin and Marcel Raymond. 4 vols. Paris: Gallimard, 1959–1969.

———. *Correspondance complète de Jean-Jacques Rousseau*. Ed. R. A. Leigh. 52 vols. Oxford: The Voltaire Foundation, 1965–1998.

Roussel, Pierre. *Système physique et moral de la femme, ou Tableau philosophique de la Constitution, de l'Etat organique, du Tempérament, des Moeurs, & des Fonctions propres au Sexe*. Paris: Vincent, 1775.

Sade, Donatien Alphonse François de. *Oeuvres*. Ed. Michel Delon. 3 vols. Paris: Gallimard, 1990.

Sauvages de la Croix, François Boissier de. *Dissertation où l'on recherche comment l'air, suivant ses différentes qualités, agit sur le corps humain*. Bordeaux: La Veuve de Pierre Brun, 1753.

Schurig, Martin. *Parthenologia historico-medica*. Dresden: Hekel, 1729.

Swift, Jonathan. *Gulliver's Travels*. Ed. Claude Rawson. Oxford: Oxford University Press, 2008.

Thomas, Antoine-Léonard. *Essai sur le caractère, les moeurs, et l'esprit des femmes dans les différents siècles*. Ed. Colette Verger Michael. Paris: Champion, 1987.

Tissot, S. A. D. [Samuel Auguste David]. *L'Onanisme: Essai sur les maladies produites par la masturbation*. Paris: Garnier Frères, 1905.

Vandermonde, Charles-Augustin. *Essai sur la manière de perfectionner l'espèce humaine*. Paris: Vincent, 1756.

Virard, P. *Essai sur la santé des filles nubiles*. London: Monory, 1776.

Virey, Julien-Joseph. *De la femme sous ses rapports physiologique, moral, et littéraire*. 2nd ed. Bruxelles: Wahlen, 1826.

Voltaire. *Mélanges de Voltaire*. Ed. Jacques Van Den Heuvel. Paris: Gallimard, 1961.

———. *Romans et contes*. Ed. Frédéric Deloffre and Jacques van den Heuvel. Paris: Gallimard, 1979.

Secondary Sources

Anderson, Wilda. *Diderot's Dream*. Baltimore: Johns Hopkins University Press, 1990.

Ansart, Guillaume. "Aspects of Rationality in Diderot's *Supplément au voyage de Bougainville*." *Diderot Studies* 28 (2009): 11–19.

Attridge, Anna. "The Reception of *La Nouvelle Héloïse*." *Studies on Voltaire and the Eighteenth Century* 120 (1974): 227–67.

Barker-Benfield, G. J. *The Culture of Sensibility: Sex and Society in Eighteenth-Century Britain*. Chicago: University of Chicago Press, 1992.

Berenguier, Nadine. "Zilia, une adolescente hors du commun." *SVEC* 12 (2004): 311–18.

Birn, Raymond. *Forging Rousseau: Print, commerce, and cultural manipulation in the late Enlightenment*. Oxford: Voltaire Foundation, 2001.

Blum, Carol. *Strength in Numbers: Population, Reproduction, and Power in Eighteenth-Century France*. Baltimore: Johns Hopkins University Press, 2002.

Bostic, Heidi. *The Fiction of Enlightenment: Women of Reason in the French Eighteenth Century*. Newark: University of Delaware Press, 2010.

Brissenden, R. F. *Virtue in Distress: Studies in the Novel of Sentiment from Richardson to Sade*. New York: Barnes and Noble, 1974.

Brookner, Anita. *Greuze: The Rise and Fall of an Eighteenth-Century Phenomenon*. Greenwich, CT: New York Graphic Society, 1972.

Carol, Anne. *Histoire de l'eugénisme en France. Les médecins et la procréation, XIXᵉ–XXᵉ siècle*. Paris: Seuil, 1995.

Carter, Angela. *The Sadeian Woman and the Ideology of Pornography*. London: Virago Press, 1979.

Cazenobe, Colette. "Le Féminisme paradoxal de Madame Riccoboni." *Revue d'histoire littéraire de la France* 88 (1988): 23–45.

Cheek, Pamela. *Sexual Antipodes: Enlightenment Globalization and the Placing of Sex*. Stanford: Stanford University Press, 2003.

Colet, Louise. *Charlotte Corday et Mme Roland*. Paris: Berquet and Pétion, 1842.

Constant, Paule. *Un Monde à l'usage des demoiselles*. Paris: Gallimard, 2002.

Cusset, Catherine. "Editor's Preface: The Lesson of Libertinage." *Yale French Studies, Libertinage and Modernity* 94 (1998), 4.

Dalton, Susan. "Gender and the Shifting Ground of Revolutionary Politics: The Case of Madame Roland." *Canadian Journal of History/Annales canadiennes d'histoire* 36 (August 2001): 259–82.

———. *Engendering the Republic of Letters: Reconnecting Private and Public Spheres in Eighteenth-Century Europe.* Montreal: McGill-Queen's University Press, 2003.

Darmon, Pierre. *La longue traque de la variole: Les pionniers de la médecine préventive.* Paris: Perrin, 1986.

Darnton, Robert. *The Forbidden Best-Sellers of Pre-Revolutionary France.* New York: W. W. Norton, 1996.

Delon, Michel. "'Ces sortes de femmes ne sont absolument que des machines à plaisir': Les Enjeux d'une formule de Mme de Merteuil." *Poétique de la pensée: Etudes sur l'âge classique et le siècle philosophique.* Ed. Jean Dagen, Béatrice Guion, et al. Paris: Champion, 2006. 341–51.

Demay, Andrée. *Marie-Jeanne Riccoboni ou de la pensée féministe chez une romancière du XVIIIe siècle.* Paris: Pensée Universelle, 1977.

Denman, Kamilla. "Recovering *Fraternité* in the Works of Rousseau: Jean-Jacques' Lost Brother." *Eighteenth-Century Studies* 29.2 (Winter 1995–1997): 191–210.

Diaconoff, Suellen. *Eros and Power in* Les Liaisons dangereuses: *A Study in Evil.* Geneva: Droz, 1979.

———. "Resistance and Retreat: A Laclosian Primer for Women." *University of Toronto Quarterly* 38.3 (1989): 391–408.

Douthwaite, Julia. *The Wild Girl, Natural Man, and the Monster.* Chicago: University of Chicago Press, 2002.

Duprun, Jean. "Sade et la philosophie biologique de son temps." *Le Marquis de Sade.* Paris: Armand Colin, 1968. 189–203.

Ehrard, Jean. *L'Idée de nature en France dans la première moitié du XVIIIe siècle.* 2 vols. Paris: S.E.V.P.E.N., 1963.

———. "Le Corps de Julie." *Thèmes et figures du siècle des Lumières.* Ed. Raymond Trousson. Geneva: Droz, 1980. 95–106.

Falvey, John. "Women and Sexuality in the Thought of La Mettrie." *Woman and society in eighteenth-century France: essays in honour of John Stephenson Spink.* Ed. John Stephenson Spink, Eva Jacobs, et al. London: Athlone Press, 1979. 55–68.

Foucault, Michel. *Histoire de la sexualité.* 2 vols. Paris: Gallimard, 1976.

———. *Abnormal: Lectures at the Collège de France 1974–1975.* London: Verso, 2003.

Gelbart, Nina Rattner. "The Blonding of Charlotte Corday." *Eighteenth-Century Studies* 38.1 (Fall 2004): 201–21.

Gilman, Sander. *Sexuality: An Illustrated History.* New York: Wiley and Sons, 1989.

Glacken, Clarence J. *Traces on the Rhodian Shore: Nature and Culture in Western Thought from Ancient Times to the End of the Eighteenth Century.* Berkeley: University of California Press, 1967.

Goldzink, Jean. *Le Vice en bas de soie ou le roman du libertinage.* Paris: José Corti, 2001.

Goodman, Dena. "The Structure of Political Argument in Diderot's *Supplément au voyage de Bougainville*." *Diderot Studies* 21 (1983): 123–37.

Gwilliam, Tassie. "Cosmetic Poetics: Coloring Faces in the Eighteenth Century." *Body and Text in the Eighteenth Century.* Ed. Veronica Kelly and Dorothea von Mücke. Stanford: Stanford University Press, 1994. 144–59.

Habermas, Jürgen. *The Structural Transformation of the Public Sphere: An Inquiry into a Category of Bourgeois Society.* Trans. Thomas Burger. Cambridge: The MIT Press, 1989.

Hoffmann, Paul. "L'Ame et les passions dans la philosophie médicale de Georg-Ernst Stahl." *Dix-Huitième Siècle* 23 (1991): 31–43.

Hulling, Mark. *The Autocritique of Enlightenment: Rousseau and the Philosophes.* Cambridge, MA: Harvard University Press, 1994.

Johnston, Guillemette. "The Divided Self in *La Nouvelle Héloïse*." *Studies on Voltaire and the Eighteenth Century* 278 (1999): 277–86.

Jordanova, Ludmilla. *Sexual Visions: Images of Gender in Science and Medicine between the Eighteenth and Twentieth Centuries.* Madison: University of Wisconsin Press, 1989.

Kadane, Kathryn Ann. "The Real Difference between Manon Phlipon and Madame Roland," *French Historical Studies* 3.4 (1963–1964): 542–9.

Kavanagh, Thomas M. "Educating Women: Laclos and the Conduct of Sexuality. *The Ideology of Conduct: Essays on Literature and the History of Sexuality.* Ed. Nancy Armstrong and Leonard Tennenhouse. New York: Methuen, 1987. 142–59.

Kermina, Françoise. *Madame Roland ou la passion révolutionnaire.* Evreux: Librarie Académique Perrin, 1976.

Kindleberger, Elizabeth R. "Charlotte Corday in Text and Image: A Case Study in the French Revolution and Women's History." *French Historical Studies* 18.4 (Fall 1994): 969–99.

Labrosse, Claude. *Lire au XVIIIᵉ siècle:* La Nouvelle Héloïse *et ses lecteurs.* Lyons: Presses Universitaires de Lyons, 1985.

Laqueur, Thomas W. *Making Sex: Body and Gender from the Greeks to Freud.* Cambridge, MA: Harvard University Press, 1990.

———. *Solitary Sex: A Cultural History of Masturbation.* New York: Zone Books, 2004.

Lee, Vera. "Innocence and Initiation in the Eighteenth-Century French Novel." *Studies on Voltaire and the Eighteenth Century* 153 (1976): 1307–12.

———. "The Edifying Examples." *French Women and the Age of Enlightenment.* Ed. Samia I. Spencer. Bloomington: Indiana University Press, 1984. 345–54.

Lindeboom, G. A. *Herman Boerhaave: The Man and His Work*. London: Methuen, 1968.

MacArthur, Elizabeth. "Between the Republic of Virtue and the Republic of Letters: Marie-Jeanne Roland Practices Rousseau." *Yale French Studies* 92 (1997): 184–203.

Marrinan, Michael. "Images and Ideas of Charlotte Corday: Texts and Contexts of an Assassination." *Arts Magazine* 54.8 (April 1980): 158–76.

May, Georges. *Le Dilemme du roman au XVIIIᵉ siècle: Etude sur les rapports du roman et de la critique, 1715–1761*. Paris: Presses Universitaires de France, 1963.

May, Gita. *Madame Roland and the Age of Revolution*. New York: Columbia University Press, 1970.

———. "Rousseau's 'Antifeminism' Reconsidered." *French Women and the Age of Enlightenment*. Ed. Samia I. Spencer. Bloomington: Indiana University Press, 1984. 309–17.

Mazeau, Guillaume. "Le Procès Corday: retour aux sources." *Annales historiques de la Révolution française* 343 (January–March 2006): 1–78. Web. 16 May 2011. http://ahrf.revues.org/9812.

———. *Le Bain de l'histoire: Charlotte Corday et l'attentat contre Marat 1793–2009*. Seyssel: Champ Vallon, 2009.

McAlpin, Mary. "Religion in Diderot's *La Religieuse*." *XVIII New Perspectives on the Eighteenth Century* 2.1 (Spring 2005): 3–15.

———. "Julie's Breasts, Julie's Scars: Physiology and Character in *La Nouvelle Héloïse*," *Studies in Eighteenth-Century Culture* 36 (March 2007): 1–20.

———. "The Rape of Cécile and the Triumph of Love in the *Liaisons dangereuses*." *Eighteenth-Century Studies* 43.1 (2009): 1–19.

———. "Innocence of Experience: Rousseau on Puberty in the State of Civilization." *Journal of the History of Ideas* 71.2 (April 2010): 241–61.

Meeker, Natania. "'I resist it no longer': Enlightened Philosophy and Feminine Compulsion in *Thérèse philosophe*." *Eighteenth-Century Studies* 39.3 (Spring 2006): 363–76.

Monstrous Bodies/Political Monstrosities in Early Modern Europe. Ed. Laura Lunger Knoppers and Joan B. Landes. Ithaca: Cornell University Press, 2004.

Morel, Marie-France. "Mme Roland, sa fille, et les médecins: prime éducation et médicalisation à l'époque des lumières." *Annales de Bretagne* 86 (1979): 211–19.

Mornet, Daniel. *Les Sciences de la nature en France au XVIIIᵉ siècle: Un Chapitre de l'histoire des idées*. Paris: Armand Colin, 1911.

Nøjgaard, Martin. "L'Education de la Marquise: Un Contre-exemple? A propos des *Liaisons dangereuses*." *Orbis Litterarum: International Review of Literary Studies* 57.6 (2002): 403–31.

O'Neal, John C. *The Authority of Experience: Sensationist Theory in the French Enlightenment*. University Park: Pennsylvania State University Press, 1996.

Outram, Dorinda. *The Body and the French Revolution: Sex, Class and Political Culture.* New Haven: Yale University Press, 1989.

Porter, Roy. *The Greatest Benefit to Mankind: A Medical History of Humanity.* New York: Norton, 1997.

———. *Flesh in the Age of Reason: The Modern Foundations of Body and Soul.* New York: Norton, 2003.

Py, Gilbert. *Rousseau et les éducateurs: étude sur la fortune des idées pédagogiques de Jean-Jacques Rousseau en France et en Europe au XVIIIe siècle.* Oxford: Voltaire Foundation, 1997.

Quinlan, Sean M. *The Great Nation in Decline: Sex, Modernity and Health Crises in Revolutionary France c. 1750–1850.* Aldershot, UK and Burlington, VT: Ashgate, 2007.

Rather, Lelland. *Mind and Body in Eighteenth-Century Medicine: A Study Based on Jerome Gaub's* De Rigimine Mentis. Berkeley: University of California Press, 1965.

Reill, Peter Hanns. *Vitalizing Nature in the Enlightenment.* Berkeley: University of California Press, 2005.

Rey, Roselyne. "La Théorie de la sécrétion chez Bordeu, modèle de la physiologie et de la pathologie vitalistes." *Dix-Huitième Siècle* 23 (1991): 45–58.

———. "Buffon et le vitalisme." *Buffon 88: Actes du Colloque international pour le bicentenaire de la mort de Buffon.* Paris: J. Vrin, 1992. 399–413.

———. *Naissance et développement du vitalisme en France de la deuxième moitié du XVIIIe siècle à la fin du Premier Empire.* Oxford: Voltaire Foundation, 2000.

Roulston, Christine. *Virtue, Gender, and the Authentic Self in Eighteenth-Century Fiction.* Gainesville: University Press of Florida, 1998.

Schiebinger, Londa. *The Mind Has No Sex? Women in the Origins of Modern Science.* Cambridge, MA: Harvard University Press, 1989.

Seigel, Jerrold. *The Idea of the Self: Thought and Experience in Western Europe Since the Seventeenth Century.* Cambridge: Cambridge University Press, 2005.

Shuttleton, David. *Smallpox and the Literary Imagination, 1660–1820.* Cambridge: Cambridge University Press, 2007.

Spary, Emma. *Utopia's Garden: French Natural History from Old Regime to Revolution.* Chicago: University of Chicago Press, 2000.

Srabian de Fabry, Anne. "Quelques observations sur le dénouement de *La Nouvelle Héloïse*." *Etudes autour de* La Nouvelle Héloïse. Québec: Editions Naaman de Sherbrooke, 1977. 19–29.

Stanley, Sharon A. "Unraveling Natural Utopia: Diderot's *Supplement to the Voyage of Bougainville*." *Political Theory: An International Journal of Political Philosophy* 37:2 (April 2009): 266–89.

Starobinski, Jean. *Jean-Jacques Rousseau: La transparence et l'obstacle.* Paris: Plon, 1957.

———. "A Short History of Bodily Sensation." Trans. Sarah Matthews. *Fragments for a History of the Human Body.* Ed. Michael Feher. 3 vols. New York: Zone Books, 1989. 353–70.

Steinbrügge, Liselotte. *The Moral Sex: Woman's Nature in the French Enlightenment.* Trans. Patricia Selwyn. New York: Oxford University Press, 1995.

Stewart, Philip. "Half-Title, or *Julie* Beheaded." *Romanic Review* 86 (1995): 36–43.

———. "Sexual Encoding in Eighteenth-Century Literature and Art." *Sexuality and Culture.* 8.2 (Spring 2004): 3–23.

Stolberg, Michael. "A Woman Down to Her Bones." *Isis* 94 (2003): 274–99.

Sturm, Ernest. *Crébillon fils ou la science du désir.* Paris: A. G. Nizet, 1995.

Sturzer, Felicia. "Epistolary and Feminist Discourse: Julie de Lespinasse and madame Riccoboni." *Studies on Voltaire and the Eighteenth Century* 304 (1992): 739–42.

Tanner, J. M. [James Mourilyan]. *A History of the Study of Human Growth.* Cambridge: Cambridge University Press, 1981.

Tanner, Tony. "Julie and 'La Maison Paternelle': Another Look at Rousseau's *La Nouvelle Héloïse*." *The Family in Political Thought.* Ed. Jean Bethke Eshtain. Amherst: University of Massachusetts Press, 1982. 96–124.

Taylor, Charles. *Sources of the Self: The Making of Modern Identity.* Cambridge, MA: Harvard University Press, 1989.

Thomas, Chantal. "Heroism in the Feminine: The Examples of Charlotte Corday and Madame Roland." *The French Revolution 1789–1989, Two Hundred Years of Rethinking.* Ed. Sandy Petrey. Lubbock: Texas Tech University Press, 1989. 67–82.

———. *La Reine scélérate: Marie-Antoinette dans les pamphlets.* Paris: Seuil, 1989.

Todd, Janet. *Sensibility: An Introduction.* London: Methuen, 1986.

Trouille, Mary Seidman. "Revolution in the Boudoir: Mme Roland's Subversion of Rousseau's Feminine Ideals." *Eighteenth-Century Life* 13.2 (May 1989): 65–86.

Versini, Laurent. *Laclos et la tradition.* Paris: Klincksieck, 1968.

Vila, Anne. C. *Enlightenment and Pathology: Sensibility in the Literature and Medicine of Eighteenth-Century France.* Baltimore: Johns Hopkins University Press, 1998.

———. "Sex, Procreation, and the Scholarly Life from Tissot to Balzac." *Eighteenth-Century Studies* 35.2 (2002): 239–46.

Walker, Lesley. "Sweet and Consoling Virtue: The Memoirs of Madame Roland." *Eighteenth-Century Studies* 34.3 (2001): 403–19.

Wellington, Marie. "Dying for Love? Three Case Studies: Prévost, Voltaire, Laclos." *Dalhousie French Studies* 45 (Winter 1998): 3–17.

Wellman, Kathleen Anne. "Physicians and Philosophes: Physiology and Sexual Morality in the French Enlightenment." *Eighteenth-Century Studies* 35.2 (Winter 2002): 267–77.

Wenger, Alexandre. *La Fibre littéraire: Le Discours médical sur la lecture au XVIIIe siècle.* Geneva: Droz, 2007.

Wilkin, Rebecca M. *Women, Imagination, and the Search for Truth in Early Modern France.* Aldershot, UK and Burlington, VT: Ashgate, 2008.

Williams, Elizabeth A. *The Physical and the Moral: Anthropology, Physiology, and Philosophical Medicine in France, 1750–1850*. Cambridge: Cambridge University Press, 1994.

———. *A Cultural History of Medical Vitalism in Enlightenment Montpellier*. Aldershot, UK and Burlington, VT: Ashgate, 2008.

Winston, Michael. *From Perfectibility to Perversion: Meliorism in Eighteenth-Century France*. New York: Peter Lang, 2005.

Wiseman, Sue. "From the Luxurious Breast to the Virtuous Breast: The Body Politic Transformed." *Textual Practice* 11.3 (1997): 477–92.

Yeazell, Ruth Bernard. *Fictions of Modesty: Women and Courtship in the English Novel*. Chicago: University of Chicago Press, 1991.

Index